JOURNEY THROUGH
THE CHAKRAS

JOURNEY THROUGH THE CHAKRAS

Klausbernd Vollmar

Gateway Books, Bath

First published in 1987
by GATEWAY BOOKS
The Hollies
Wellow, Bath, BA2 8QJ

© 1987 by Gateway Books

Reprinted 1988, 1989, 1992

First published in German in 1985
as *Fahrplan durch die Chakren*
by Werkstatt Edition, Axel Dietriech Verlag

Translated by John Button

Set in Century Book 10½ on 11½

Printed and bound in Great Britain by
BPCC Wheatons Ltd, Exeter

British Library Cataloguing in Publication Data:
Vollmar, Klausbernd
Journey through the chakras: exercises
for healing and internal balancing.
1. Chakras (Theosophy)   2. Exercise
I. Title
613.7   RA781
ISBN 0-946551-42-1

Contents

Acknowledgements		1
Foreword		5
1.	Yoga for Westerners	17
2.	Body Exercises and the Holographic Concept of the Human Body	25
3.	The Chakras in Different Cultures	37
4.	A New Approach to the Chakras	53
5.	The Individual Chakras	69
	The Base Chakra/Muladhara	72
	The Sacral Chakra/Svadisthana	75
	The Navel Chakra/Manipura	77
	The Heart Chakra/Anahata	80
	The Throat Chakra/Vishuddha	81
	The Third Eye/Ajna	85
	The Crown Chakra/Sahasrara	88
6.	Deciding Which Chakra to Work On First	91
7.	Red Tantra: A Digression	93
8.	The Exercises	97
	Physical Exercises/Asanas	97
	Breathing/Pranayama	98
	The Mind	101
	Therapy	103
	Preparing for the Exercises	104
	Some Final Tips	105

9. Exercises for the Seven Chakras   107
    The Base Chakra/Muladhara   107
    The Sacral Chakra/Svadisthana   113
    The Navel Chakra/Manipura   120
    The Heart Chakra/Anahata   128
    The Throat Chakra/Vishuddha   133
    The Third Eye/Ajna   139
    The Crown Chakra/Sahasrara   142
10. Exercises for All or Several of the Chakras   145
11. Conclusion   150
12. Bach Flower Remedies in Chakra Work   153
    Glossary   161
    About the Author   167

Illustrations

FIGURES

Fig. 1 The Chakras and their Locations on the Hands and Feet — 27

Fig. 2 The Chakras and their Location on the Human Skull — 28

Fig. 3 The Chakras and the Corresponding Reflexology Points — 36

Fig. 4 The Location of the Minor Chakra of the Right Hand — 43

Fig. 5 The Celtic Cross — 61

Fig. 6 The Spine Seen from the Back with the Locations of the Five Lower Chakras — 73

Fig. 7 The Five Lower Chakras as a Pentagram — 84

Fig. 8 St George and the Dragon — 121

TABLES

Table 1 The Chakras in the System of Elements — 44

Table 2 Everything You Ever Wanted to Know About The Chakras — 56

Table 3 The Planetary Resonances of the Chakras — 70

PHOTOS

Photographs of the exercises for the individual chakras appear between pages 109 and 138 alongside the description of the exercises concerned.

Acknowledgements

This book could not have been written without the help, criticism and discrimination of the participants in my yoga groups and workshops.

My particular thanks to my teacher, Dr von Ungern-Sternberg, who with humour and wisdom led me deep into my inner self, showing me where East and West meet to celebrate their links. Then there is the shaman, Black Horse Chavers, who helped me on my way with love and understanding, and who taught me to explore the shadows of my soul with the clear light of truth.

Many other people have helped me enormously, even though some of them never think of themselves as being spiritual. They have taught me not to become rigid in my spirituality, to come back to earth when I was in danger of losing touch completely with the real world. Only your behaviour in everyday life shows whether you have truly integrated the lessons of chakra work.

It was during several visits to Findhorn, a twenty-five-year-old New Age community in northern Scotland, that my eyes and heart were opened to the full

realisation that every person and every situation
provides a useful lesson. It is important to be open to
these teachings all the time, even when it feels
uncomfortable. With this new awareness I have found an
alternative to the traditional moralistic and patriarchal
image of God: God is not a personification of our guilt,
but a spirit present in every situation, everything, and
everybody.

I would also like to thank Barbara Widdup, Uschi
Schuch and Wolfgang Altmann, who have never been
able to hold back their criticism and have sometimes
argued passionately with me — thank God, they still do!
They know I can be a difficult friend, and that I
sometimes inhabit a different world which they find
hard to comprehend. They have showed me that love is
able to bridge even the biggest differences, and that if
we can avoid preaching and proselytising, wonderful
creativity can result from the juxtaposition of apparent
contradictions. I am also grateful to Barbara and to
John Button for their help and cooperation in preparing
the English version of this book.

Last but not least I want to thank my 'men against
sexism' group in Solingen, especially Manfred Flöther
and Frank Wengenrodt. They helped me to find my self-
confidence, gave me the courage to act as an individual,
and showed me my limits and inhibitions.

When I started to write this book, in sunny autumn
weather on the north coast of Norfolk, I asked myself
how much I wanted the material in it to come from the
collating, assessing and integrating of other people's
work, and how much I wanted it to be my own. In the
end it is hard to say where one ends and the other
begins. All I know for certain is that there is never
anything which is completely new, and that I must be
eternally grateful for whatever it was that led me to
undertake this exploration, and for the many aware

people I met on my travels. The impetus for the journey has taken me to many places and many cultures, and has brought me safely back to the peace and tranquility of a little English village by the sea.

I hope the exercises included in my book bring you the same sense of peace and tranquility.

Klausbernd Vollmar
Cley-next-the-Sea, May 1987

Foreword

This book stems from my own experience with yoga and the techniques of humanistic psychology. During most of my training in chakra work I have had no teacher or guru, but I have had a great deal of contact with other people who regularly practise yoga and other forms of bodywork.

Like many other people, I almost drowned in a wave of therapy en route from the student movement to an understanding of spirituality, and during the sixties anarchism influenced me in such a way that I am only now learning to accept a teacher.

But a certain anti-authoritarian attitude is often just as important as the acceptance of a teacher. In order to deal responsibly with authority, both from others and within oneself, it is necessary to live with the contradiction.

The Polish author, Gyorgy Doczi[1], has coined the term 'dinergy'[2] for any growth-giving energy which is based on opposites. I have noticed again and again in my life that in conflict situations I tend to take sides in the

hope of making my life easier, the price of which has
often been the loss of creativity and happiness. It took
me a long time to realise that it helps me more to let
the tensions created by such conflict situations to
continue and to live through them, thereby transforming them into a creative spiritual energy. Only by
letting tensions work inside you can creative energy be
set free, and the often simplifying intellect be
transformed into intuition.

Those people who, in a difficult situation, do not
immediately act or respond, but who allow themselves
the time and space to let tensions work within themselves, create the potential to deal responsibly from
their inner selves. This is what yoga is all about.

I see yoga as a creative link between tension and
relaxation, effort and release.

How do you work with your tensions? What do you do
with them?

Try making a list of the tensions you feel at the
moment, for example:

    loneliness versus independence

    self-confidence versus the need for recognition.

One of things I would like to do in this book is to ask
you, the reader, continually to ask questions of yourself,
particularly if you have already had some experience of
yoga.

Every spiritual search, including that of yoga, depends
upon constant questioning. The refusal to question
leads to rigidity, and makes all our efforts futile,
because experience gained through yoga will no longer
be able to reach our heart. or soul.

Knowledge and uncertainty are complementary qualities, just like good and evil, yin and yang. If one becomes
dominant this causes an imbalance; routine and boredom set in, and movement, liveliness and the creative
dance around the point of equilibrium become lost.

This book presents many practical exercises and ideas to help you experience the energy centres in your body, and to feel the energy flowing throughout your body. Try not to be limited by any ideas you may already have about yoga or chakras. They often only confirm what you already know. It is important to trust your own experience rather than concentrating on preconceived ideas, concepts and techniques, otherwise you run the risk of becoming like the astronomer who spent all the time reading the star charts and never looked at the sky. In freeing yourself of concepts and structures, these exercises may well lead you into new realms of experience.

All the exercises presented here can be done without a teacher; you alone are responsible. Don't be frightened by the possibility of making so-called mistakes; mistakes too have creative potential and can lead to new realisations. Remember that in this age of computers and data processing the ability to make mistakes is an important human privilege!

Though the exercises in the book can be done without a teacher, the book itself is a sort of authority, and this is yet another paradox. But the best teacher is always your own inner voice. I would like to help you to become aware of that inner voice, so that you can do what your body tells you to. This is very easy to say, but it needs considerable time and commitment. You cannot learn to do chakra yoga in half an hour. When you really get into these exercises you will start to find yourself doing chakra work in your everyday life — at work, while you shop or cook a meal, at the discoteque or while you make love. It isn't that you would have the exercises permanently in your mind — that would be awful. It means that you would be living your yoga, seeing the whole of your life and surroundings in a new way.

Working with the chakras is more to do with
consciousness-raising than with physical exercise,
yet as long as you don't get too attached to them
the physical exercises can often give you an indication of different states of consciousness. "Don't
get attached" — the first lesson of the Buddha
Sakyamuni.

If while you do the exercises you feel that you need a
teacher, you will almost certainly find the right person
because you will be in a state of awareness that will
attract what you need. Don't worry about it.

Working with a teacher does have certain advantages:
you have to learn to listen to someone else, and you
have an opportunity to work out your problems about
authority figures. But remember that you can learn
from everyone you meet. Everybody you meet can be
your guru, and of course you will always have your own
inner guru. Again, don't worry about it.

If you want to explore beyond the exercises in
this book and think you need a teacher, always ask
yourself what you expect from a teacher. Can you not
give this to yourself? What is stopping you helping
yourself?

While I was working on my throat chakra I found
myself getting stuck even though I worked very hard. So
I went to a teacher and worked with her for several
months. Eventually I discovered that I needed to
accept the hurdle, and that it was by looking at
acceptance that I made progress. Having accepted that
I went on alone, since she could help me no further.
Before long the block in my throat disappeared, my neck
relaxed, and I found I could breathe more freely.

I now live in the countryside, and my great teachers
are nature and my garden. I see in the plants, shrubs and
trees similar growth processes to my own. In my garden
shed hangs a poem of Goethe:

There is always in nature
Something which demands respect.
It is not wholly within us,
Nor yet wholly outside us,
But we grasp it without reserve,
This sacred yet open secret.

Flower blossoms grow in spirals from their centres; the shapes of growing plants have perfect proportions. There is always a certain tension between the plant and its surroundings, and I like to think of the formation of the leaf of a plant as a similar process to the development of a part of a person's character. Proportional growth is a subject I have often considered; growth both in relationship to ourselves and to our surroundings.

When I look at yoga movements, particularly the chakra exercises, I often see the same geometrical forms as those of plants. While the spiral of growing starts inthe centre of the plant, most of my yoga exercises start at the 'os sacrum' — literally 'the sacred bone'. The movements of my hands often reflect what is going on in the rest of my body; here the centre point of the movements is the wrist.

If you open your hand, then put your thumb and first finger together and hold the other three fingers out as straight as you can (the gesture of concentration and teaching), the movement creates the same logarithmic spiral as do plants, snails, and the spiral nebulae in the heavens.

When you practise yoga you will become aware of the geometry of your body movements, the lines, circles and spirals that reflect tension and relaxation in your natural surroundings.

In our culture geometry has always been a means of approaching self-knowledge and higher awareness. The tradition began in Classical Greece, and was continued by medieval cathedral builders and the brotherhood of

the Freemasons. This is reflected in the traditional
symbols used by the alchemists for body (□), mind
(△) and spirit (○), a symbolism also used in yoga:
□   representing   asana,   △   meditation,   and   ○
pranayama.

I have been influenced by the Swiss psychologist Carl
Jung, who took a critical view of yoga in the West.
Reading Jung and undergoing Jungian dream analysis
have given me the confidence to adapt yoga and chakra
exercises to make them relevant for Westerners today. I
therefore follow no particular classical school, theory or
ideology.

It is paradoxical that yoga and chakra work are so
important and serious that we can only explore them in
a childlike, playful way. Playing connects us with our
deep childhood roots when movement and creativity
were inseparable, and when reflection and difficulty
rarely intervened. The German classical poet and
philosopher Friedrich von Schiller says in his aesthetic
writings: "Human beings are only human when they are
playing".

Play, concentration and seriousness do not exclude
each other, and working with yoga, tantra and chakras
in a playful way, modifying them as we need to, prevents
us from becoming soulless technicians of the discipline.

I have always had problems with the idea of 'work',
especially in such combinations as 'chakra-work' and
'body-work'. Marx was right when he said that work
needed to be redefined to distinguish it from the
alienating work that so many people do, but I wonder if
such a redefinition is possible in a culture so tied to the
existing notion of 'work'.

I strongly believe in the principle of hope. If a growing
number of people in our society can experience their
bodies, minds and spirits positively, then perhaps the
rest of humanity will experience that energy too. The

British biologist Rupert Sheldrake[3] suggests that everywhere in the world is a field of experience. This 'field of experience' is intersected by different 'morphogenetic fields', so that living organisms partake of the experiences of others even though they may have no direct contact with each other (for anyone who knows about quantum physics, this is the biological equivalent of Bell's Theorum).

Neo-Einsteinian physics teaches that each part of the universe is always everywhere, so we must take into account the fact that events which appear to be unconnected are in fact connected, though in a non-causal and non-localised way.[4]

To put it simply, everyone who works with the chakras helps everyone else who is on the same path, and is in turn helped by everyone who is working (or has ever worked) in this way. Everybody changes the course of yoga in their individual way; thus yoga remains alive and relevant, not a dead museum piece.

On a smaller scale, this interconnectedness can be experienced in every yoga class. When I practise yoga and chakra work with friends, a synergetic energy is created which aids concentration and helps me to work in a more aware and precise way than I can achieve when I am on my own.

I should also mention that my academic training is in classical clinical psychology and humanistic psychotherapy. I bring this psychological and intellectual background into my chakra work too. There is a psychological dimension to all human behaviour.

However, I do want to avoid 'psychologising' everything. My heart knows that on our human journey from the animal realm to the gods we consist of much more than our psyches alone. I like to see human beings as an integration of body, mind and psyche.

Classical psychology is a very young science, and

humanistic psychology, born from the discomfort with our times and our society, is even younger. Yoga is by comparison an ancient science (really more of a lifestyle) which deals especially with the process of human individuation.

During my training as a psychotherapist I found that Western psychology loves disease, the pathology of human suffering. I find this preoccupation with illness very negative, ignoring as it does the unnecessary dualism of 'health' and 'illness'. Yoga and the philosophy of chakra work are based on the idea that every human being is perfect just the way they are. Sadly, most people find this philosophy impossible to relate to.

Since Maslow, Fromm and Janov, humanistic psychology has attempted to move towards this positive concept, yet many humanistic practitioners (and their clients) are still locked inextricably into the 'illness' model of human existence. I have been in many a group where I was accused of being naive and unrealistic for suggesting that everybody (including me!) was absolutely fine the way they are. In bioenergetic groups I have been told that the ongoing battle with my 'character armour' ('persona' in Jung's terms) was all that was important[5], and my 'rigidity' in believing in the perfectness of people has been attacked. I think both yoga and psychotherapy have their value, but only in yoga have I felt complete acceptance, and acknowledgement that I am basically sane and healthy.

In the shift from the Age of Pisces to the Age of Aquarius our need for a spiritual dimension to our lives has become increasingly pressing. Pisces (a water sign) indicates the importance of feelings; Aquarius (an air sign) the importance of mind and spirit. Seen from this perspective we can understand the contribution of humanistic psychology without seeing feelings as the

ultimate aim in life, and recognise that we cannot
practise our spirituality without acknowledging the
importance of feelings. It would be nice if the freeing of
our feelings could serve a spiritual aim.

I know I have been quite hard on humanistic psychology, and of course it has its uses. Which of us is
completely in touch with our feelings and can express
them without anxiety? By the end of the Age of Pisces
we should have learned to integrate our feelings with
our spirituality: the mark of the New Age, the Age of
Aquarius. We should make the most of living through
the exciting times of the transition from one age to
another, integrating everything we have already learnt.

How can we make the links between the emotional
work and the spiritual work?

In meditation the spiritual and emotional work
become one. Meditation often gives us clues about our
past (this is called 'Pratiprassav' in the yoga
scriptures), and we can use this insight to help solve
problems in the present. Once the insight has been
brought to the surface using yoga and meditation,
techniques of humanistic psychology (bioenergetics,
gestalt or whatever) can be used to work with it.

I often find my understanding blocked by the preconceptions and assumptions of psychotherapy. At
times like this I have to remember that 'having fixed
ideas is being against God'.

But does yoga really not have any fixed ideas? I
believe that yoga and humanistic psychology can
complement each other in a fruitful combination of
East and West. And thus we arrive back at the idea of
dinergy.

Some more thoughts about humanistic psychology.

I have difficulty accepting the insistence of humanistic psychology upon regression to pre-rational levels
of human development. Ken Wilber[6] stresses that

body-centred therapy often has a very regressive
tendency, leading the client into pre-personal,
cultistic and narcissistic channels. Mind you, yoga as it
is practised by many Westerners can be criticised in the
same way — its adherents assiduously avoid any
intellectual reflection and enjoy their time spent in an
Eastern fantasy-world where all is love and light.
'Don't think!' they say, followers of yoga and humanistic practitioners alike rejecting our intellectual
heritage. I agree with Freud's analysis that this leads to
pathological and regressive separation.

Despite all its innovations, humanistic psychology
still tends to cling to the mechanistic medical tradition
that mind is somehow a physical function of the body. I
believe that every experience can be examined
intellectually — to be able to explain is an important
aspect of being human and to avoid explanation is to be
immature. Psychoanalysis is just as important as
bodywork and sensitivity games. Coming as I do from
the angle of yoga, I have to see these techniques in the
round, and part of any integrated approach to humanistic psychology must be to ask what the purpose is of
this search for feelings.

What I particularly like about both humanistic
psychology and yoga is their stress upon perception, and
their emphasis that perception always comes before
thought.

People who practise yoga because they are frightened
of therapy, scared that their feelings might overpower
them, are strongly advised to go into therapy before
they start yoga, and certainly before they start chakra
work. The form of therapy is not vitally important —
gestalt, bioenergetics and rebirthing can all be very
succesfully integrated with yoga and chakra work, since
they all share similar ideas about the flow of energy in
the human body.[7]

There I conclude the introduction. Perhaps your expectations have already changed. Perhaps you are clearer now, perhaps disappointed. Whatever your reaction, if you are ready to continue our exploration I invite you to tune into the spirit of yoga, the spirit of the here and now.

1. Doczi, G. *The Power of Limits* Shambala, U.S.A., 1981.

2. 'Dinergy' is based on two Greek words — 'dia', on the other side, and 'energia', energy. 'Dinergy' thus means literally 'the effect of the difference': this is what I want to express here.

3. Sheldrake, R. *A New Science of Life* Blond and Briggs, 1981; Paladin, 1983.

4. Dossey, Larry *Space, Time and Medicine* Shambala, U.S.A., 1982. In 1964 the physicist Bell produced a proof that all events are interconnected, even if they have no obvious connection in space and time. This is a consequence of quantum theory, and the counterpart of Jung's notion of synchronicity.

5. A typical example of the 'disease model' of humanistic psychology is the beginning of Wilfried Teschler's book on polarity therapy: *The Polarity Healing Handbook* Gateway Books, 1986.

6. Wilber, Ken *Up From Eden* Doubleday, USA, 1981; Routledge, 1983.

7. There are clear parallels between the Reichian concept of orgone energy, the prana energy in rebirthing, and the prana energy in the yoga scriptures. The 'field theory' of gestalt therapy comes close the the 'here-and-now' philosophy of yoga.

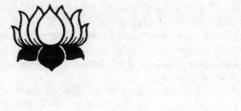

1
Yoga for Westerners

*"Psychoanalysis itself, and the string of techniques
that has arisen from it — surely a peculiarly Western
development — is the effort of mere beginners when
compared to the state of the art in the East."*
Carl Gustav Jung

If we do yoga and chakra work, the first question we
need to ask ourselves is how far we should suppress and
sublimate our own selves as we follow the path of
spirituality.

I suppose that the aim of every path — be it a
spiritual path like yoga or a therapeutic one provided by
humanistic psychology — is to make contact with our
true self, and thence to make connections with other
people's true selves. Making the link with your own
true self opens up the connections with the wider
world. In the moment that you make contact with the
real you, the whole universe opens up and suddenly you
find that there is no 'inside' and 'outside'. Can we
really encourage this experience of connectedness by

using a particular method, however simple or detailed it might be?

Is there not a danger that we might limit the abundance and complexity of the cosmos by using a particular technique, or suppress important aspects of the self which need to be explored?

Even if we have our doubts about suppression, surely sublimation can lead Westerners towards creative achievement. It may be useful to stop at this point and ask yourself why you have chosen to look at the way of yoga rather than the many other ways that are available. Is it possible that the way of yoga and chakra work can help to break a person's unconscious structures and destructive patterns — their 'neuroses' as Freud called them?

Let me try and explain what I mean by giving some examples.

Among the many strands that make me who I am there is one side of me that wants to be in control, wants to tell everyone how things ought to be. This control mechanism is a result of my fear of surrender, the anxiety of letting go. Chakra work can all too easily strengthen this need to control, and I have to be careful.

A highly disciplined Westerner who chooses the way of yoga always runs the risk of identifying totally with yoga and its exercises, and thus limiting rather than freeing themselves. As Jung says:

"Westerners do not need to learn superiority over nature, neither their own nature nor nature as a whole. They have both forms of control perfected almost devilishly. What Westerners do not have, however, is a conscious humility in relation to nature — both inner and outer. What they need to learn is that they cannot always do what they want. If they do not learn this, then their own nature will destroy them. They cannot hear the soul which revolts against this suicidal tendency.

"Because they turn everything into techniques, everything that is not obviously a technique appears to be dangerous, is destined to fail. Practising yoga for your health is as useful for a Westerner as any other form of exercise, but yoga is deeper than that. If I understand it correctly, yoga aims to achieve much more — no less than the liberation of the consciousness from its attachment to all objects and ideas. You cannot free yourself from what you cannot comprehend, so the Westerner must first explore those objects and ideas. This is what we in the West call the unconscious"[1]

This exploration of the unconscious seems to me to be all-important. Returning to my example, a disciplined Westerner who decides to practise yoga is in danger of using yoga and chakra work as a way of blocking the path to the unconscious, thus creating yet more rigidity. If this happens it is virtually impossible to use the yoga exercises to achieve liberation.

Not without good reason is the highest aim in yoga called 'the white light'. White light contains all the colours of the rainbow as seen through the prism of yoga. In some yoga systems the opening of the highest chakra — the thousandfold lotus or 'sahasrara' — is symbolised by the rainbow, thus expressing the idea of multiplicity as the combination of contrasting (complementary) colours.

Now let us look briefly at aggression, a real challenge to positive thinking. Is aggression inappropriately-expressed love, or is it an important power for change, or is it simply energy in the wrong place?

Aggression has its linguistic roots in the Latin *aggredi*, which means 'to come closer'. People who practise yoga and chakra work often think of aggression as evil, bad and negative.

When I am feeling aggressive I can no longer control my breathing in a disciplined way. I cannot concentrate on relaxing my muscles. But is that bad? What is this multiplicity of feelings really all about?

Later I will describe some exercises relating to the manipura chakra (the Japanese 'hara', the centre of gravity of the body) and explain the concept of 'positive fighting', an important element in shamanism. If we believe that yoga should somehow 'rise above' aggression, is there not the danger of misunderstanding the cultural roots of yoga and becoming demoralised? For 'morality' is alien to the essence of yoga, or at least it is to the Buddhist school of yoga which stresses direct experience and understanding (almost akin to the scientific method) rather than morals. At some point — when you start to work with your navel chakra if not sooner — you will need to ask yourself what you mean by aggression.

What you believe to be aggression, and whether you see it as good or bad, is determined by your culture and background. What do you understand by 'aggression'? Can you identify positive aspects of your aggression?

I spoke before about the basic idea of yoga, and whether there was in fact a basic idea. There is a general belief in all yoga texts that people should be good, and should think and act taking the welfare of both themselves and others into account. Apart from this general ideal, yoga scriptures tend to avoid dogmatism, believing that the way of true liberation is not to lay down strict guidelines — which for many Westerners is a difficult concept.

Can you understand the contradiction?

It may puzzle you that the first spiritual exercise of yoga is to recognise that the quiet laziness of acceptance is a dangerous starting point. Everything —

as Albert Einstein has pointed out — is relative to the observer. Thinking itself makes everything relative, and does thinking and the use of the intellect not affect all human behaviour? I always think that mind is a manifestation of spirit and spirit a manifestation of mind; both mind and spirit are manifest in the physical body — the living body.

The path of yoga is systematic — at least when seen from the surface. First you train your body so that you can sit motionless; then you can control your breathing. With this controlled breathing you can then control your emotions. You can then learn to meditate and watch your mind.

Yet everything is connected; every particle contains the whole. Thus the spirit contains aspects of mind and body; the mind aspects of spirit and body. To put this holographically[2], if we want to distinguish mind within the mind-body-spirit continuum, the distinction is also reflected at the level of body and spirit. While working with the chakras you always work on all levels at the same time, so it is not particularly important whether you work specifically with the mind, the body or the spirit.

Why then do we continue to find the hierarchy of body, mind and spirit taught in yoga classes? Such a hierarchy is never found in the ancient Asiatic scriptures.

By now you may be thinking to yourself how intellectual all this is, shaking your head and about to close the book. We shall move to the practical exercises very soon, but since it is such an important part of our academic tradition, it is important to put the intellect in its proper place. You should always understand what you are doing in your yoga, but without resorting to pretentious theorising. You should feel free to criticise, and be prepared to deal with the paradoxes which affect and move you.

And yet another paradox: you should never follow any path which says 'you should'. This is crucial to chakra work.

How you ever stopped to ask yourself why we Westerners always want to change ourselves? Why can we not be content with being the way we are? For me yoga contains both aspects — the element of change and the acceptance of who we are. This reminds me of the cycle of the Tarot: in the beginning is the Fool, and after moving through twenty-one changes he ends up again as the Fool.

Thinking and talking about yoga in this way involves us in different levels of language, corresponding with different levels of consciousness. The classical Greeks used to differentiate between 'logos', the language which expresses the interrelatedness of objects, and 'mythos', the language of nature and the unconscious.

The structure of logos is based on logical and accurate reasoning, and expresses itself within the laws of cause and effect. The structure of mythos is iconographic or pictorial, and often illogical and dreamlike. The difference between logos and mythos is reflected physiologically in the difference between the right and left hemispheres of the brain, and the right and left sides of the human body.

Each language cannot be translated into the other; thus yoga cannot be understood in a logical way. But it is nevertheless important to try, and we can at least discover the limits of rational language and reasoning. Yoga, however, always goes further.

I believe that yoga and chakra work go even further than humanistic psychology in offering possibilities for the liberation of feelings in a creative and spiritual way, though humanistic psychology can be used very effectively by Westerners as a first step on the path of yoga.

Finally in this chapter I would like to give you some advice about meditating on yoga and power.

In my yoga classes I often ask the participants why they want to practise yoga and work with their chakras. Most people say: so I can become a better person. In such responses I often detect an unconscious striving for power — maybe because I know that striving all too well!

Another paradox: Maybe if we could see power in everything, then power would dissolve like smoke in the wind. I am convinced that using power in an unconscious way can be very dangerous, because when it is unconscious it is uncontrolled. If I cannot see my power clearly, I cannot decide clearly whether or not to use it.

Chakra work has a very systematic aspect, and all systems include an element of power. I have often asked myself whether yoga is therefore a very patriarchal male discipline.

In this age of adventure holidays we can go to places where we can brave the elements, display our courage, and win against all the odds. Maybe the hero doesn't ride quite like John Wayne any more, but he is just as effective at conquering new worlds, the last remaining frontiers of space and time.[3]

Before you start working with the chakras — as you should with any spiritual discipline — clarify your attitude towards power. If you cannot find aspects of power within yourself, be extremely careful. How are your ego trips?

There are no clear and straightforward answers to these questions, but it is vitally important to raise them. Put the other way round: asking the right question or asking the question in the right way is in itself to have found the answer. Once you set out on the

path of yoga and chakra work you will find many
questions which have no simple answers.

But there is much more to life than finding the right
answers.

It is said in Zen that that a question addressed in the
right way is itself the answer.

1. Jung, Carl Gustav *Yoga and the West* Collected Works Vol.
11, Routledge, 1978.

2. For more about the holographic aspect of the human body
see the next chapter. This whole book is based on a
holographic concept of the universe.

3. This is where Einstein and the Tibetan lama share the
same path. In Tibetan mythology the land beyond the border
is seen as a vast formless land; the world on this side of
the border is called 'samsara' — the illusion.

2
Body Exercises and the Holographic Concept of the Human Body

"Yoga is neither sitting in the lotus position nor looking at the tip of your nose. Yoga is the oneness of the soul and the cosmic mind."
Kularnava Tantra

In this chapter I want to emphasise the holographic aspects of chakra work for the Westerner. Chakra work must be understood in terms of its essence, not simply be seen as an alienated system of physical exercises.

Many books and workshops dealing with the chakras tend to concentrate on chakra work merely as a technique involving a series of exercises, but I want to begin with the idea of oneness: "One is a good place to start the number system, but it is a wretched place to end it. 'All is one' has become such a cliché among lazy intellectuals that it must be stressed that the web of life contains plurality as well as oneness, endless diversity as well as connection."[1]

This game of oneness and diversity! The harmonic proportions of all the measurements of the body are

25

repeated in the different limbs. The feet, the hands and
the head all provide a microcosm which mirrors the
macrocosm of the whole body. The same can be said
about body, mind and spirit: the body reflects the
structure of the mind and the soul, and the mind
reflects each of the other two qualities. It is because of
this 'enfoldment' that we are able to say that we
create the way we are. But what does this enfoldment
of the whole in every part of the body really mean?

When you explore what we have in common, you
cannot distinguish between human beings and nature
without losing important aspects of awareness. This
loss always creates alienation, drawing you away from
oneness, concentrating on one aspect of the self at the
expense of the others. This disharmony in turn disturbs
the whole body. The form and structure of the whole
body are hidden in every limb and organ, and a change in
one tiny part can be detected both in every other part
and in the whole.

A hologram is a three-dimensional picture in which
every element of the picture contains the whole
hologram. The information of the whole picture is
contained perfectly yet individually in every part
(figures 1 and 2 indicate how this works within the
human body).

The concept of the hologram is at least as good a
model of the human body as the model of 'oneness'.[2] It
mirrors exactly what the yoga sutra of Patanjali says
about human beings in a metaphorical way. Here is part
of the second century Buddhist Avatamsaha sutra:

"It is said that in the sky of Indra is a net of pearls so
arranged that when you look at one pearl, you see all
the other pearls reflected in it; whenever you enter
one part of the net you set a bell ringing which
reverberates from every part of the net, from every
part of reality."

The holographic view is not new. It can be found in

Figure 1
The Chakras and their Locations on the Hands and Feet

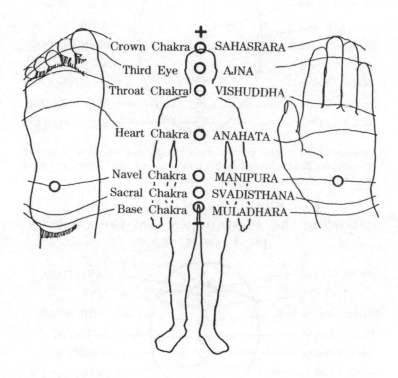

This illustration shows the points in the hands and feet which, given light pressure or massage, can stimulate the chakras. The stimulation of these points stimulates the healing potential of the relevant chakra.

Figure 2
The Chakras and their Location
on the Human Skull
(seen from above)

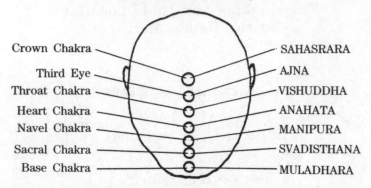

You can find these points most easily if you first find the Sahasrara Chakra, which is projected on to the highest point of the skull, directly above the spine.

The Skull of a Newborn Child
Showing the Fontanelles and the Chakras
(seen from above)

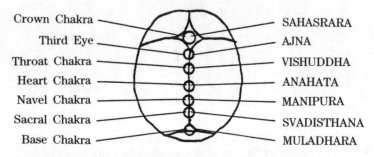

This illustration, which shows the fontanelles as well as the chakras, may help you to locate the chakras on the skull.

the Kabbalah in the symbol aleph, and in the seventeenth century *Monadology* of the German philosopher Leibniz. What is new, however, is that we now have the means actually to produce holograms. Dennis Gabor (1900-1973) described the basic theory of holography in 1947-48, but until the development of lasers in the 1960s it was impossible to create a hologram. Holography has both a technical and a theoretical aspect, the latter rapidly becoming a universal theory based on quantum mechanics. A fascinating aspect of the theory is the recognition of the 'hidden variable' — the fact that the observer is always part of the system being studied, thus demolishing the myth of the independent scientific observer.

When the holographic principle is applied to the human body, it is clear that chakra work involves us with every aspect of the body. We cannot become limited by one particular technique, fixated on a method which corresponds precisely with the lack of soul in our environment, and a tendency which contradicts the very essence of yoga. Unless you use the energy of your soul, you cannot activate or open a single chakra.

I have used this word 'soul' several times, but what I really mean by it cannot easily be expressed in words. Think of it instead as a symbol — the symbol of soul or spirit is a circle, a blue circle.

Throughout this book I will be suggesting body exercises, but every exercise should bring you in touch with your feelings and with your mind. Feel free to wander between them and try not to be limited by any of them.

Yoga exercises can only be properly integrated if you explore yourself exactly as you are. Lack of integration in yoga can easily lead to frustration, tension and boredom. When I talk about 'integration' I mean the thorough working through of experience at all levels, body, intellect and soul all playing a vital part.

So, never work with the body exercises alone; it makes it difficult to experience the body as a whole. Listen to your body, watch your mind, and notice your feelings . . .

All at the same time . . .

Each contains all . . .

In yoga we mostly work with and on the spine — in Tibetan metaphorical language the spine is called 'meru', the mountain. The aim of the exercises is a straight spine.

Most of us have a crooked spine — 'crooked' meant both physically and metaphorically. Our spine can show us a complete picture of our physical development from conception to the present. Accumulated in the spine is our personal history, the history of the human race with all its changes and emotions. How can we differentiate between history, physiology, and deep beliefs?

In its connection to the others, each vertebra enfolds the wholeness of all these aspects. Whenever we move our spine the elements begin to dance, a movement that can lead to liberation.

What is liberation for you . . .?

Liberation from what . . .?

Liberation to what . . .?

When we are ready to open ourselves to the communication of our spine, every aspect of the body can be stimulated at the same time. There is no body posture ('asana' in yoga) which does not affect our mind and our emotions, yet there are disciples of yoga who are not aware of these links, and who are unable to open their bodies to this sense of wholeness.

If you do not feel any emotions while you are doing the exercises, if no sudden thoughts cross your mind, the chances are that you are blocking yourself from seeing and understanding the communication within your body.

You can either use yoga exercises as a technique for suppression and sublimation, or as a path of liberation. The choice is yours.

The degree of alienation and lack of connectedness within our society is reflected in some schools of yoga, where the new initiate could be forgiven for thinking that yoga consists of nothing more than a series of physical and breathing exercises, followed by a short meditation.[3] It is hard for Westerners to imagine how naive some yoga schools are when it comes to their basic theory.

On the other hand, if we try to see what is intimately interconnected in a purely analytical way, we are in danger of thinking negatively, and being out of line with the synthetical perspective of yoga. I tend to think of 'seeing' in terms of analysis, since whenever we focus on something we only see part of the whole. The whole picture is provided by an expanded consciousness. The purpose of yoga is to lead us to this wholeness, and to open up its healing power to us and to our society.

Few Westerners have ever thought about the morality of chakra work and yoga. Maybe the experience of yoga is too individual to consider the wider moral issues — chakra work, after all, deals with the individual, not with the masses. Yet we also live at a time — the much-mentioned Age of Aquarius — in which more and more Westerners are turning to Eastern wisdom. There are thousands of evening classes in yoga, and quite a number of people now know something about the chakras — which in ancient times were after all a secret wisdom. This is why it is a particularly important time to think about why we choose this particular path.

If we cannot see chakra work as a way into our psychological structure, if we do not connect chakra work with our spiritual energy, then the current boom in yoga will lead us not to healing, but into ego trips, rigid discipline, the ethics of consumerism, and perverted personal behaviour.

The opportunities provided by chakra work link mind, body and spirit together indivisibly. Yoga makes it possible to experience the true relationship between the universe, humanity, the single cell and the individual body.

After such a lot of theory, let us now try an exercise from the movement therapy of the the Israeli practitioner, Moshe Feldenkrais. This exercise may help you to tune into the experience of oneness:

Stand up straight and place your right hand on your back. Swing your left arm and bend your upper body first down, as though bowing deeply, then back up to the left. Follow the movement through so that your left hand touches your right shoulder. Now stand up straight again and relax. Move your head freely as you do this exercise, and keep your eyes open.

Where was the centre of movement in your body during that exercise? What shapes did you create in the space that you worked in? Now do this exercise several times with your left hand on your back and your right arm swinging. Can you tell any difference between your right (male) side and your left (female) side? Were you aware of the space around you? Where are the boundaries between you and the surrounding space?

Now sit with your spine straight (maybe on a chair, though it is better not to be supported by the back of the chair, or in the lotus position on the floor). Sit for at least ten minutes and listen to your body.

Did you feel any tension in your spine? If so, where? Can you hear what your spine is telling you?

Most people in our culture experience tension between the third annd fourth dorsal vertebrae (at about the level of the heart chakra). This often indicates a tendency towards egocentrism, and means that the person is not flowing, is not trusting that life will provide them with everything they need to be happy. This tension of the heart chakra — often called a closed heart chakra — is connected with a particular reflexology point on the sole of the foot, two finger-widths in from the highest point of the instep. You can find this point yourself. Even if your heart chakra is wide open, you can feel it; it is more sensitive to pressure than the area all round it. When you think you have found it (not before!) look at Figure 3 at the end of this chapter.

This all-too-common tension of the heart chakra can sometimes be felt as a slight bending of the spine, and it needs to be treated at both a physical and a spiritual level. If you only treat it on the physical level (using reflexology or massage, for example), all you will succeed in doing is moving the tension somewhere else in the body — often a place where it is much harder to treat it. On the other hand, if you try to straighten your spine by pure willpower you will probably do more harm than good, tensing all the muscles in the spine, including the antagonists[4], and putting the vertebrae — especially their outer surfaces — under unnatural pressure.

So what can you do?

Working only on the physical level to straighten the spine only creates more intractable tension elsewhere (your ego trip simply finding another place to escape to). Well, here is your chance to think of dis-ease as a challenge, and to listen directly to your tensions, inhibitions and limitations.

Tense the area around your heart where you feel discomfort when you do the heart chakra exercises

(see Part 4 of the chapter on the individual chakras).
Feel where your heart is, and breathe deeply and
regularly into this point. Notice the emotions that
come up, and they will show you (though maybe not
immediately — have patience!) where the deeper
reason for the tension lies. Follow your feelings and
gradually let them become stronger. Now stay with
them — to run away from them now would simply be
defensive. Observe your feelings carefully, so you can
think about them later.

If after a month or two of working in this way you do
not feel any change, then it is probably a good idea to
drop yoga for a while.

The first changes are usually experienced as a difference in the quality or location of the pain — it may
move its position, or become stronger or weaker, or
apparent only when you tense yourself. When the pain
starts moving, it usually disappears fairly soon afterwards. If the pain or tension stays in the same place and
feels much the same, you might think about trying some
bodywork, such as bioenergetics or rebirthing. Both are
quite compatible with yoga in terms of their ideas
about energy. These techniques will probably help the
feelings come to the surface and erupt, whether it is to
do with fear, pain, hatred, grief, or whatever else you are
holding on to. Whatever the feeling, expressing it will
free your body.

If it is only a temporary tension you may be able to
breathe it away using the 'bhastra' technique (which is
rather like the rebirthing technique of breathing in and
out without taking a break between breaths), and use
prana energy alone as your therapist, freeing your
tensions simply by breathing them away. The purpose of
the exercise is not to work hard at expressing your
feelings; if you are doing the breathing properly the

feelings will arise quite involuntarily. Trust yourself! What are the mental attitudes and ideas that you want to change? Always be aware that yoga and meditation can be quite dramatic when it comes to the release of 'dark' feelings which have been resisted for many years.

This approach to tension in the body illustrates clearly the holographic aspect to human body. The body seen holographically deserves therapy of the same quality.

All physical tensions are the result either of too little energy (too much 'yin') or too much energy (too much 'yang'), and illustrate the delicate balance between yin and yang in the way we live our everyday lives. It might help you to look at your birthchart at this point. Look at your seventh house and see which planets you have in the sign of Libra.

Temporary tensions can also be dealt with by using reflexology, and Figure 3 shows how the chakras are projected on to the foot. To reach the chakras, you need to massage the appropriate areas with a considerable amount of pressure. I always use my thumb.

To conclude this chapter I would recommend meditating on the Tarot card number XVI — The Tower. There you willl find the archetypal symbol of the dangers of power and technique alienated from spirit.

1. Leary, Timothy *The Game of Life* Ronald, U.S.A., 1973.
2. In this book I shall use 'hologram' and 'wholeness', and 'holistic' and 'holographic', as synonyms.
3. This practice is part of the 'hatha yoga' tradition in India, Tibet and Nepal, but it has little to do with chakra work as it is practised in the West. Always remember the enormous cultural differences between Asia and Europe.
4. 'Antagonists' are the muscles that work in opposite directions.

Figure 3

The Chakras and the
Corresponding Reflexology Points

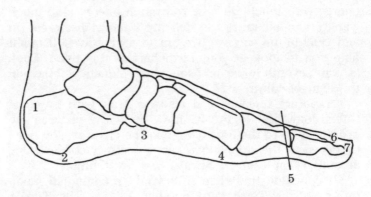

1. Base Chakra   MULADHARA
2. Sacral Chakra   SVADISTHANA
3. Navel Chakra   MANIPURA
4. Heart Chakra   ANAHATA
5. Throat Chakra   VISHUDDHA*
6. Third Eye   AJNA
7. Crown Chakra   SAHASRARA

* This point seems to vary from person to person, but is always found on the same part of the foot.

3
The Chakras in Different Cultures

All cultures have some concept of chakras as energy centres within the human body. Look at the saints of Christian tradition — there is the halo painted in filigree gold, symbolic of a person who has opened their Crown Chakra, the thousandfold lotus, to the heavens. What is the tonsure of monks if not a reminder to work with the highest chakra, the positive pole of the body? Are the carvings of spirals and snakes in Celtic stonework, found from Ireland to the Iberian peninsula, from Scandinavia to Malta, a reminder of the Kundalini serpent of Hindu mythology? Do they indicate a knowledge of the pulsating life energy in nature and in the human body?

We find the snake again in the Biblical story of the Fall. According to the sagas, the Merovingian kings who ruled over large areas of France and Germany at the time of King Arthur were high masters in the use of chakra energy. They were even referred to as yogis, and were skilled in the use of magic. The skulls of the Merovingian kings show a small artificially-drilled hole at the point of the Crown Chakra, exactly like those found in the skulls of early Tibetan monks.[1]

Documents and sagas about the Merovingian kings say that they had amazing healing powers. They were said to be clairvoyants and to have telepathic powers. Who knows what is fact and what is fiction? But their skulls have survived, and sure enough they all have a hole drilled at the Sahasrara Chakra.

We find similar holed skulls from Egypt, from the time of the construction of the great pyramids, though in Western literature they are usually seen as proof of 'medical surgery'.

It seems that there has been knowledge of the energy centres in the body in many different cultures, and the Crown Chakra appear to be the most important. This is symbolised today in the crowns worn by kings and queens.

For Christians and Sufis[2], the Heart Chakra has come to be the most important today. Medieval literature — Wolfram von Eschenbach's *Parzifal* for example, or Manichean song manuscripts — shows clear evidence of knowledge about energy centres in the body. There is evidence from every culture that at least those people who were initiated into the ancient wisdom knew about the body's energy centres, and worked with them. If you want to find out more about this tradition, read the history of the Albigensians (the Cathars) and the Knights Templar, or study the alchemical literature.

A very interesting book which shows the parallels between the Asiatic traditions of chakra work and the beliefs of the Cathars and the alchemist tradition is Miguel Serrano's *El/Ella* (He/She): *The Book of Magical Love*.[3]

Since Leadbeater wrote a classical study of the chakras, the chakra teachings have been taken up by theosophy, and anthroposophy, which has partially grown from theosophy, has developed his ideas into a more or less complete theory of the chakras.[4,5]

Madame Blavatsky was right to warn against the use of chakra work to produce 'mesmeric phenomena', as she called them. She was describing a sort of magnetism, an attraction which can easily be used to very selfish ends. Alexandra David-Neel[6] gives a vivid and gruesome account of this sort of misuse of knowledge about body energy in the form of the 'bon' practices in Tibet at the turn of the century, showing clearly how the power of chakra work can be subverted to the evil ends of black magic.

The Anthroposophist approach to the chakras is very ambiguous. With a certain prudery they warn against working with the lower chakras — meant more in a moralistic sense than a locational one! — especially with the Sacral Chakra (Svadisthana). They recommend that students of the chakras should concentrate solely on the upper chakras, which is a very idealistic approach.

I find this very worrying, since such an attitude towards the human body all to easily provides the rationale for a new and limiting moralism, reflecting the fears of our culture. Every human being is also a sexual being, and sexuality and creativity are closely connected with each other.

At the same time I see the danger of a great rift in society, between those who are fixated on sexuality and those who refuse it completely. It is very important to work with the sexual chakra (the Sacral Chakra, Svadisthana), because the aim of all chakra work is integration and harmony between all the different aspects of the person.

Only a sexually fulfilled human being is able to send positive energy back into the world. Tantric literature, especially in the West, tends to stress the transcend-

ence of sexuality. This can be a dangerous limitation to
the vital expression of life energy, which can easily lead
to dis-ease. If, on the other hand, the transcendence of
sexuality is not forced, it can be very beneficial.[7]

In Hatha Yoga, and particularly in its Tibetan form,
sexual abstinence is demanded from the very beginning.
If you study this form, you must understand that it
involves complete isolation from the world; in fact the
final initiation involves being immured for a period of
three years, three months and three days. What we in
the West call 'yoga' could hardly be more different. And
yet Hatha recognises the balance of male and female
energies in union — Ha-tha itself means 'sun and
moon'.

After so much text we need another exercise,
otherwise all the energy will be bound up in our heads.
Now we need to bring it down into our bodies again to
balance it.

> Stand up straight and become clearly aware of the
> floor under your feet. Place your feet slightly wider
> apart than the width of your shoulders, and let your
> arms fall relaxed by your sides. Touch your thighs with
> your hands — right hand on right thigh, left on left.
> Now focus on a point straight ahead of you and,
> breathing in, push your pelvis as far backwards as it
> will go. Now breathe out, thrusting your pelvis as far
> forward as you can. This exercise is designed to
> ground yourself and to express your male sexual
> energy. Do it for one or two minutes, concentrating
> on any resistance you may observe, on any pain, on
> your breathing, on the messages your body may be
> trying to tell you, on your thoughts about what a
> stupid exercise this is. Now lie down on the floor on
> your back, as relaxed as possible. Watch your feelings
> and the flow of energy through your body.

How do you feel about your male aspect?

Now let us try the female counterpart of that exercise. Because we all posses qualities of both animus and anima, we always do both exercises together.

Stand up straight again, your feet slightly closer together this time, about the width of your shoulders apart. Bend your knees slightly, and let your arms hang loosely by your sides. Now roll your pelvis to the right, so you make a circular movement parallel to the floor; after a while change directions and circle your pelvis to the left. Breathe regularly, and try to synchronise your moving and your breathing. Again watch for any resistance, be aware of your breathing and the rhythm of your movements. Do this exercise for one or two minutes, then lie down on your back again and relax.

When you breathe in you take in energy; when you breathe out you can feel the energy rising in your spine and falling through the front of your body.

Can you feel the energy centres in your body?

Are there points where you feel the flow of energy more clearly?

How do you deal with the female side of your sexuality?[8]

These easy exercises show how easy and natural it is to be able to feel the energy centres in the body. They do not necessarily have to be the precise points where the charts say your chakras should be located — descriptions of their exact locations differ enormously anyway. Try to free yourself from any preconceptions you may have about where you think your chakras should be! Some people say there are 88,000 chakras in the body — what does that really mean? It means that if you are sensitive enough, you can experience every point of your body as an energy centre. This was perhaps what Sigmund Freud meant when he said that every part of the human body was an erogenous zone. It's a nice idea, isn't it?

But we live in a culture where the importance of the chakras has been increasingly overlooked, and they now have little place in our ideas about health and healing. Freud rightly called ours a culture of desensitisation and sublimation.

When I talk about the chakras, I am usually referring to the seven main chakras, though whenever these seven chakras are activated, you are in fact activating the whole body.

The inside of your hands (see Figure 4), and the knees and ankles, are also important energy points — the so-called 'minor chakras' — even though I do not deal with them in detail. You can experiment with them yourself, working with them and understanding them. You will find this easy if you have already worked with the main chakras.

The two minor chakras in the palms of the hands are particularly important for healers — spiritual healers in the Philippines, for example, work extensively with these chakras.[9]

To summarise: anyone who is in touch with their body will be able to feel their energy centres in one way or another, especially in the period of relaxation after the stimulation of the chakras. It comes as no surprise, therefore, that the concept of the chakras is found in every culture.

I like to visualise the chakras as an archetypal pattern of spirals of energy within the human body, mirroring the energy spirals of the planet. The symbolism of the spiral is found throughout mythology, in legends and fairy tales — as water wheels, spinning wheels, whirlpools and serpents.

Figure 4
The Location of the Minor Chakra
of the Right Hand
(seen from the inside of the hand)

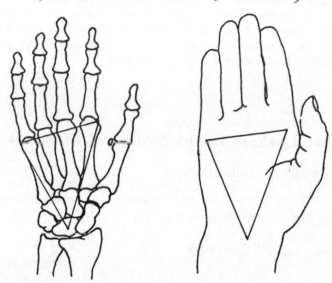

The bones of the right hand

In Christian times the pagan practice of working with the energy centres in the body became equated with the work of the devil. The devil, seen as a fallen angel, was initiated into the wisdom of energy flows.

One of the most recent ideas about chakras is based on the new physics, and sees chakras as reservoirs of 'prana' at different capacities — 'prana' being the basic kind of body energy, the energy that binds the psyche to the body.[16]

This rather mechanistic model is based on the idea that the chakras (the reservoirs) which have more prana,

at a different level of vibration, tend to be more open.
The frequencies of vibration, or concentration levels,
increase from ether to earth, and thus the different
chakras are connected with the elements. Sahasrara and
Ajna are at such low concentrations that there is no
known element which connects with them. It is in the
upper chakras that the psyche and the physical plane
have the least connection — in the language of physics,
there is the lowest level of coupling.

Table 1

The Chakras in the System of Elements

Crown Chakra	SAHASRARA	⎫ lowest density	field of	
		⎬ of prana	consciousness	
Third Eye	AJNA	⎭		
Throat Chakra	VISHUDDHA		field of communication	
Heart Chakra	ANAHATA	air △	field of emotions	yang
Navel Chakra	MANIPURA	fire △	field of power	
Sacral Chakra	SVADISTHANA	water ▽	social field	yin
Base Chakra	MULADHARA	earth ▽	field of activity	

As well as the links between the chakras and their specific elements, I also find it useful to think of their links with the realms of nature. In our Base Chakra and its quality of earth we find ourselves in the mineral realm — the first of the nature realms. With the Sacral Chakra and its watery quality we are in the plant realm; with the Navel Chakra at the centre of the body and its fiery qualities we make contact with the animal realm and its untamed wildness (a wildness which is still, fortunately, within each of us). With the heart chakra we become human beings under the influence of mind and the quality of air — take note that the quality of being human comes with the heart chakra! The throat chakra has links with the ether, the base from which all the other elements arise, and which gives us a glimpse of the level of mastery that can come with an understanding of the last two chakras — the Third Eye and the Crown Chakra.

What I want to do now is look very briefly at the range of ideas about chakras which have appeared in other books. There are really only very few books worth reading on the subject, since other authors have in general merely copied their ideas and thoughts from them.

One of the most interesting books on the chakras, suitable as an introduction to the subject from the alchemical point of view, is that by the organised and concise author Peter Rendel.[10] Anyone who likes a systematic introduction will enjoy this book, which is based on Hindu chakra theory.

The outstanding work on the chakras from the Asiatic point of view, based on the original texts, is that by Arthur Avalon — an Arthurian pseudonym for Sir John Woodroffe, who became a disciple in India of Laya Yoga. In my opinion he provides the best specialist information about the ancient Indian wisdom of the chakras. This classic, much quoted but unfortunately seldom read, is called *The Serpent Power*.[11]

Arthur Avalon wrote two other books on the same theme — they are both as hard to read as *The Serpent Power*. His books are filled with Sanskrit theory, and one of Avalon's greatest achievements is to translate every idea very accurately into Western concepts. Avalon was the first Western student of the chakras to equate Eastern ideas with Western analogies, for all his overwhelming detail and complexity in explaining Laya Yoga (a form of yoga which concentrates on the chakras). He describes the complicated exercises in a way that can only be done if you have studied closely with a teacher. If you study Avalon's *The Serpent Power*, you will notice that he constantly draws parallels between chakra work and Western ideas about individuation. His choice of pseudonym shows that he saw the connection with Celtic beliefs about self-discovery — Avalon, the Celtic paradise, the island where King Arthur found healing, Arcadia.

In the end it is not important which path you follow on the journey of self-discovery. While you can learn a great deal from looking to the East, you should never forget your own traditions — this is exactly what 'Arthur Avalon' is trying to remind us.

Another interesting book about the Hindu concept of the chakras has been written by the Indian artist Harisch Johari.[12] Here you will find useful analogies, but not so much information. On the other hand, it is the only book I know of which looks at the chakras from an artistic point of view. It is a painting book for adults, developed from a workshop run at the Thorwald Dethlefsen Institute in Munich in 1975. Unfortunately, Johari has very conventional ideas about art, and does not see the connection between free artistic expression and chakra work. I believe that chakra work can be expressed very creatively in abstract art forms, particularly using Goethe's theories about colour.

In 1980, together with a friend, I led a workshop in southern Germany on art and free expression. Each member of the group meditated in front of large white canvas (about four feet square), and at the sound of a gong each participant took their brush, chose a colour, and painted one unbroken line on the canvas, before returning to meditate on the canvas. Later we connected this exercise with meditation on the individual chakras, concentrating on the colours which were important for each person. Just at the moment, while typing this passage, I sense my Throat Chakra as being bright red — after a few days I expect it will return to its more usual blue!

The forms and colours used in a free artistic meditation of this kind are a far more dynamic expression of chakra energies than conventional Hindu chakra paintings, but as a Westerner I find them much more useful. Yet I also enjoyed colouring in the black and white drawings at the end of Johari's book, and I learned a great deal about Hindu concepts of chakras in the process.

In an informally-written book by Anand Margo[13] you will find a fascinating mixture of the ideas of Bhagwan Shree Rajneesh — who himself studied Tantra — and the ideas of the Arica group, of which John Lilly and Claudio Naranjo are important members. What is made very clear in this book is the connection between chakra work and the methods of humanistic psychology, from rebirthing to the experience of the isolation tank.

From a Theosophical point of view, C.D. Leadbeater is the author of the classic book *The Chakras*.[14] Leadbeater worked closely with Annie Besant, who was one of Madame Blavatsky's closest co-workers, and who enjoyed debating the role of Asian wisdom and

esoteric Christianity with Rudolf Steiner. Unlike the
ancient sources of Laya Yoga, Leadbeater only recognises the Spleen and Navel Chakras in the lower part of
the body. He doesn't recognise the sexual chakra — the
Sacral Chakra; to him it is part of the Base Chakra. A
result of living in the culture of Victorian England?

His book contains a large number of tables, diagrams
and illustrations, and shows the chakras as coloured
spirals. The West German clairvoyant, Franz Wenzel,
sees the chakras in the same positions and colours as
Leadbeater; this is interesting, since clairvoyants
generally seem to have their own individual colour
coding for the chakras, and see the auras of the same
person in quite different ways.[15] Maybe this similarity is
due to Wenzel's anthroposophical background — what
you believe will inevitably colour even your psychic
perceptions.

The colours and auras of the chakras do not remain
constant, of course. Any meaningful colour chart can
only concern itself with the analytical and theoretical
aspects of colour within the spectrum (see Table 2).

A completely different but no less inspiring book
about the chakras for modern Westerners is Inhoffen's
Yoga Book.[16] The author of this book is an engineer
working in electronics, and he explores the Tibetan form
of chakra work from the point of view of the new
physics. Using well-chosen scientific analogies, he
explores prana energy, the chakras, and the rising of the
kundalini energy (or 'nadis' as it is properly described).

I found his excursions into scientific psi research
rather on the level of anecdote where yoga is concerned.
I found it difficult to take his notions seriously when he
talks about UFOs being immortal yoga masters.
Apparently the UFOs radiate energy according to the
chakra energy levels of their pilots.

One of the best yoga books is that by Marcus Allen.[17]

The theme of the book is that 'love opens the heart and the senses', and the book teaches how to work with that energy, using affirmations. It explains the history and philosophy of Tantra very clearly and concisely, and at the same time gives many practical hints and exercises.

And last but not least, there is a very important book by Oscar Marcel Hinze called *Tantra Vidya*[18], a Hindu expression for the study of the web of creation. For me this book provides a very important and extensive historical and astrological study, the most important cornerstone for the holographic study of Tantra and the chakras.

I have asked myself quite often why a man like Sir John Woodroffe would write such a detailed book about the raising of the kundalini, knowing that it could only be achieved successfully with the help of a responsible teacher. Perhaps the function of Woodroffe's book about the serpent power is to provide a guru in the shape of a book.

Would it be possible to raise your kundalini safely after reading his book? Surely not. Is it indeed responsible to write books like this about such dangerous spiritual paths?

Books like this seem to be written mostly to help one's own 'inner guru', and you need first to make contact with this, the best of teachers. Your own inner guru should hold you back from moving along the path too quickly. This is not always the case, however, as is shown clearly by the work of the Spiritual Emergency Network (SEN) in Big Sur, California, where a group of doctors and transpersonal psychotherapists helps people who have had spiritual accidents.

This collection of books will probably give you all the information you need, but if you are particularly interested in the subject, Avalon's *The Serpent Power* has a splendid bibliography. If you are particularly interested in the Indian concepts of the chakras, then Bagchi's *Studies in the Tantras* mentions a lot of the important literature.[19]

If you are looking for the important Tibetan sources of chakra yoga, I will mention just the most accessible: Lama Anagarika Govinda's book about Tibetan yoga.[20]

The original Tibetan writings are virtually impossible to get hold of, and for very good reasons, since so many very powerful teachings are described in such a necessarily metaphorical way. These teachings can enable a human being to transform absolutely anything about their life as they progress along the road towards enlightenment — as long as they are used for the welfare of all living beings.

1. See Baigent, M.; R. Leigh and H. Lincoln *The Holy Blood and the Holy Grail* Cape, 1983.

2. The Sufis have similar concepts to the Buddhists and Hindus. They call it 'the immensity'. See Corbin, Henri *The Man of Light in Iranian Sufism* Shambala, U.S.A., 1978.

3. Serrano, M. *He/She* Routledge, 1973.

4. Leadbeater, C.W. *The Chakras* Theosophical, U.S.A., 1972.

5. Steiner, Rudolf *Knowledge of Higher Worlds: How is it Achieved?* Anthroposophic, U.S.A., 1977.

6. David-Neel, A. *Love Magic and Black Magic.*

7. A sensitive book dealing with these issues is Elizabeth Haich's *Sexual Energy and Yoga* Allen and Unwin, 1972.

8. You will find this exercise again, though with minor differences, in the section on the Svadisthana Chakra.

9. Meek, George W. *Healers and the Healing Process* Theosophical, U.S.A., 1978.

10. Rendel, Peter *Introduction to the Chakras* Thorsons, 1979.

11. Avalon, Arthur *The Serpent Power* Dover, U.S.A., 1976.

12. *Das große Chakra-Buch* Freiburg, 1979.

13. *Tantra: Weg der Ekstase* Meinhard, 1983.

14. See footnote 4.

15. Weigel, Giesela and Franz Wenzel *Die entschleierte Aura* Forstinning, 1983.

16. Inhoffen, H.v. *Yoga* n.d.

17. Allen, Marcus *Tantra for the West* Whatever, U.S.A., 1977.

18. Hinze, Oscar Marcel *Tantra Vidya* Freiburg, 1983.

19. Bagchi *Studies in the Tantras* Calcutta, 1939. In the 1930s many books were published in India about Tantra and the chakras, mostly in English.

20. Govinda, Anagarika *Tibetan Yoga and Secret Doctrines* London, 1935.

4
A New Approach to the Chakras

*"Thus the superior man acquaints himself
with many sayings of antiquity
and many deeds of the past,
in order to strengthen his character thereby."*
I Ching

Most descriptions of the chakras start by constructing a model or diagram — in fact this chapter started life being called 'A Model of the Chakras' — but even at best models can only provide a glimmer of the wisdom contained in chakra yoga.

This is true of many symbolic systems: in astrology, for instance, Mercury symbolises the speed of the intellect, though he is characterised as the messenger of the gods. Mercury, the principle of the intellect, provides order and explanation, yet he himself is no god, no important piece of the model.

If we want to make contact with these important elements, with the gods, then the models of chakra work with their mercurial character can only help to

point the way. But they are not the thing itself. So it is
with all the following concepts about the chakras: they
are only tools to help you make contact with your own
energy centres.

Anybody who has read books about the chakras will
have come across the idea that in the depths of the
base chakra sleeps a snake-like creature called
Kundalini, which can be awoken using special exercises.
After maybe twenty years of discipline, you can reach
the mysteries of Raja Yoga, where you can work with
the Kundalini within all your chakras. These ideas are
based in beliefs about Kundalini energy which are totally
alien to Westerners; very few people in the West are
able or willing to put so much time into yogic practices.

There is also a description of a beautiful girl who lives
in the Muladhara Chakra, and who climbs your spine if
you practice certain exercises.

These are all very mechanistic concepts — a snake
rises, a girl climbs up your spine — but they are of
course only metaphors which allow us to describe
energy movements which we cannot express clearly in
any other way.

I neither know nor care whether the Kundalini really
rises or not, and I am not particularly interested in
detailed discussions about the right and wrong ways to
make the Kundalini rise. I think that intellectual
discussion of any sort is ultimately the wrong way. We
must obviously include the psychological dimension in
our chakra work, but we must not get stuck on
mechanistic and physiological models.

We must understand Kundalini energy as but one
name for the creative power of the universe that lives in
everyone.

The physical side of the chakra work is important, but
it is only one aspect of the work, and tends to be overly
stressed by the materialistic West — probably partly

because it is the most easily accessible aspect, and also because racy stories about what happens when the Kundalini is awakened have given rise to wild speculations. The vision of being literally burnt by the heat of a Kundalini which has been raised wrongly is a dangerous and exciting prospect for anyone who sits behind a desk all day in the depths of boredom. I suppose it makes for gripping headlines, creating as it does a unique blend of horror and adventure.

At the possible expense of disappointing you, I must admit that I do not believe that the Kundalini literally rises. If you are being honest, don't stories like this frighten you? Fear is the greatest enemy of self-understanding, and of chakra work — fear is both compulsive and addictive.

Trust your body. If you listen to it carefully it will tell you where to to go, and when to be careful, when to slow down or take a break.

We tend to attract what we fear the most. Fear can be painful, but it does give us the opportunity to look deeply into ourselves. By dealing with our fear we can learn a great deal about ourselves. The important thing is not to be controlled by fear.

I see the seven chakras as symbolising the seven evolutionary ways of approaching life. This corresponds with the way of the Fool in the Tarot, or the cycle of the signs of the Zodiac from Aries through to Pisces. Each of the seven chakras is associated with particular experiences, challenges and opportunities. For Westerners the chakra work is a concrete way of finding your true self, a way which is connected directly with the way you live your daily life.

To help you understand this concept I have set out Table 2 to show the analogies and correspondences of the different aspects of our lives in relation to the seven chakras.

Table 2
Everything You Ever Wanted to Know about the Chakras

Chakra	Mantra	Element	Part of Body	Endocrine Gland
SAHASRARA Crown	Aum	(light)	higher brain, right eye	epiphysis
AJNA Third Eye	Aum	(spirit)	lower brain, left eye, nose, ears	hypophysis
VISHUDDHA Throat	Hang	Akasha = ether	**mouth**	thyroid
ANAHATA Heart	Yang	air	**penis**, heart, circulation, lungs	thymus
MANIPURA Navel	Rang	fire	**anus**, stomach, liver, gall bladder	pancreas
SVADIS-THANA Sacral	Vang	water	**hands**, muscles	gonads
MULAD-HARA Base	Lang[1]	earth	**feet**, spine, nails, teeth	adrenal

Temperament	Lesson	Therapeutic effects	Breathing
master	Unification of the higher and lower self[3]	senility	
enlightened	intuition, overcoming nihilism	tension, fear, bad dreams, glandular disturbance	pause after breathing in
awake	real communication, integration, peace	disturbance of thyroid, depression, speech problems	pause after breathing in
melancholic	service, overcoming distance, hatred, restlessness	angina pectoris, circulation problems	breathe without pausing
sanguine	mastery of desire, power, ambition	diabetes, cancer, whooping cough, indigestion	breathe without pausing
choleric	surrender, release of what cannot be digested	urogenital problems, arthritis, oedema, etc.	pause after breathing out
phlegmatic	release, grounding, overcoming suffering	calms the central nervous system, tension in the spine, sexual problems	pause after breathing out

	Sense	Colour	Astrology[5]	TAROT Pingala	TAROT Sushumna
SAHASRARA		purple	Virgo/ Pisces	the sun	the universe
AJNA		violet	Gemini/ Sagittarius	the tower	the moon
VISHUDDHA	hearing	blue	Leo/ Aquarius	death	the devil
ANAHATA	touch	green	Aries/ Libra	fortune	the hanged man
MANIPURA	sight	yellow	Taurus/ Scorpio	the chariot	the hermit
SVADISTHANA	taste	orange	Cancer/ Capricorn	the emperor	the lovers
MULADHARA	smell	red		the magician	the empress
				ACTION Asana	UNDER-STANDING Meditation

| TAROT | POLARITY | | | |
Ida	Female	Male	Stones	Deities
judgement	neutral		diamond, onyx	the duality of animus/anima is transcended
the star	+	–	coral, zircon	Param-Asiva, Hakini
temperance	–	+	topaz, carnelian	Ardana-Resvara, Sakini
strength	+	–	ruby	Isa, Kakini
justice	–	+	jade, sapphire, pearl	Maharudra, Lakini
the heirophant	+	–	emerald	Vishnu, Rakini
the high priestess	–	+	emerald	Brahma, Dakini

LOVE
Pranayama

In this table you will find all the correspondences that I shall discuss when we come to look later at the individual chakras.

First, however, I want to look at the Tarot, because I believe that it shows most clearly how we can understand the chakras as a way of living our everyday lives.

In order to make the links with the chakras, I have separated the twenty-one cards of the Major Arcana into three groups; thus each chakra is associated with three cards. In the first column is an indication of what in Tantra is called the yang way, the way of the male sperm. This path, from The Magician to The Sun, symbolises the relationship of the active male energy with the energies of the seven chakras.

In chakra work we always start with the lowest chakra, and there we find The Magician, the archetype of the man who goes out into the world, tries to understand the laws of nature and the laws of society, and acts accordingly. This represents the materialistic way of dealing with life — the manipulation of the environment. The Magician creates his own space in life. In a sense we are all magicians and are more or less successful in the role. Every woman also has this aspect deep within her, if not already experienced then still waiting to be freed.

The next step on the male path leads to The Emperor, at the sexual or Sacral Chakra. The Emperor has to produce a son — King Arthur's challenge. He has to act creatively and responsibly without destroying his links with his society.

After the materialistic way of approaching life, we now come, via the way of creative social action, to The Chariot, associated with the Manipura Chakra. Here the man succeeds despite all obstacles — but is the victory a real one? Does everything really go according to plan? The Chariot is represented as a wagon drawn by two sphinxes, one black and one white. Is it really possible to keep the light and dark aspects of yourself in perfect balance, or will the chariot tip over? Tension and relaxation must be in perfect balance — this is the Japanese concept of the Hara.

The male path now goes on to The Wheel of Fortune or The Wheel of Life. We have now reached the level of development of the Heart Chakra, and the associated circulation and movement of the heart. Now you need to learn the laws of movement and how to work with, rather than against them. Until you can learn to stand at the still point of the axis you will always be turning with the wheel, though you cannot fully understand this until you reach The Sun, or the Sahasrara Chakra.

Before you reach that point you have to master the step of communication, associated with the Throat Chakra. Here is the link between feeling and thinking, a difficult step which involves the death of the old personality.

Then you must master the level of the Third Eye. When you have an understanding of this level you can let go of the need for models and systems. Now you can experience The Sun in yourself. This is symbolised by the Celtic Cross, in which the sun shines from the centre. The cross symbolises the body, and the circle symbolises the sun shining out from within the body.

Figure 5
The Celtic Cross

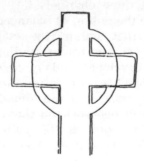

This way was developed from its Celtic origins by the
tradition of esoteric Christianity, which flowered in
places like Iona and Lindisfarne.

This then is the way through the chakras seen from
the point of view of 'doing' — the male or yang way. In
the physical ideas of Laya Yoga this path is called the
Pingala channel.

For me each of the three sets of Tarot images also
corresponds to one of the three paths through which
the Kundalini should rise. Pingala — the channel of
action — corresponds with the Asanas — the physical
aspect of yoga. Ida is the channel of love, the female
path which is connected with Pranayama — the
breathing aspect of yoga. This path lifts our emotions,
quietens them, and brings us peace. In Tantra this is the
way of menstrual blood. The third channel is the so-
called Middle Way. Called Sushumna, its channel is the
spine. I sometimes think of it as being associated with
suffering, but you might like to meditate on this before
agreeing with me. This channel is also associated with
meditation, and in Tantra it is the path of sexual
intercourse — Maithuna.

When we see Pingala, Ida and Sushumna in association
with the three aspects of yoga — Asana (bodywork),
Pranayama (breathing) and meditation, it is easy to see
why it is believed that the Kundalini should rise equally
through the three channels.

Alongside the notion of balanced rising energies is the
implication that action (the male aspect), love (the
female aspect), and understanding (the central aspect)
need to be developed equally. Real development cannot
occur without any of these three. And we have to
develop our male and our female sides, just as Jung
emphasised in his work on the animus and the anima.

Let us now look at the path of love through the
chakras, the Ida aspect. You might like to do this

yourself by meditating on the Tarot cards and the aspects of the path which they represent.

Lay out the seven Tarot cards in the order I have suggested and look at them. See what associations, feelings, thoughts and images come to you. Let it become clear to yourself that there is no real growth without love.

Now sit comfortably and feel your heart beating. Close your eyes, and meditate on the following five aspects of the path of Ida:

love

mercy

joy

serenity

humility

Now you might like to look at the cards of the path of Ida again, all the time being aware of the beating of your heart. Can you feel your heart?

At the level of the Muladhara Chakra — where the male Magician stood — is his counterpart The High Priestess. These two images complement each other — The Magician wants to understand the secrets guarded by The High Priestess — this is the meaning of the Veil of Isis. The High Priestess guards the mystery within yourself (a reflection of the mystery of the world) — if you cannot approach this mystery with humility then you are not yet ready to start the chakra work. If, however, you can love both yourself and others, you can move up the path of love, symbolised by a pale green moon, from the passivity of the Base Chakra and the image of The High Priestess to the more active way of The Hierophant. Both The High Priestess and The Hierophant have the power of initiation that is based in love.

Do you love yourself? Can you, at least sometimes, love other people more than you love yourself? Here, at the level of the Sacral Chakra, ask yourself whether you can surrender to yourself. This leads to the more general question: Can you let yourself into your real self?

From here we move to the archetype of Justice. How do you deal with power, with ambition, with your will? At the level of the Manipura or Navel Chakra it is important not to overstress success.

How do you deal with your wants and your desires?

Do you lose touch with your spirit when you are successful?

If you have integrated all the lessons of your life up tonow, you will know the power of your heart. In the Tarot pack created by Aleister Crowley and Frieda Harris, this archetype is called Desire.

Power and Desire; Desire or power?

From the perspective of depth psychology, this is the opportunity to free yourself from your mother, to open up your capacity to love both yourself and others.

If you have already gone through this process (and here it is important to be aware of your dreams, even if you do not fully understand them), then you need to learn how to express your love appropriately. The lessons of the Throat or Vishuddha Chakra can help, providing the healing powers of artistic expression — the art of healing.

You may even reach the level of the Third Eye or Ajna Chakra in this lifetime. Here you will find the archetype of the star within you, remembering that "everybody is a star"[4] in unity with the cosmos — a white light from the darkness of the universe. Some sages speak of 'impersonal love', and it is worth meditating on this idea.

Finally we reach the resurrection, The Last Judgement — what the Buddhists call Amithaba, or formless beginning.

But the Sahasrara Chakra is not really the end. There is no end to the growth process, and there are many levels which we have no awareness of as yet.

Many people ask where we go when we have reached this level. How do we go back again? The answer is that the experience of the higher levels will remain with us, but there are always new lessons to be learned at every level. Zen teaches that 'when you reach the top of a mountain, just go on climbing'.

Something which is repeatedly emphasised in Tantra is that when you have learned to work with the higher chakras, you will be able to step outside yourself. You will be able to identify fully with the exercises and lessons of all seven chakras, and yet be able to step outside yourself as well. This is yet another of the paradoxes of every path of self-discovery.

Why are there seven steps on this path? Why seven chakras? Physiological explanations alone are hardly sufficient; at the very least the physiological level is reflected on the mental level.

Rudolf Steiner sees the development of the human being from birth to death as a series of seven-year periods, reflecting the Biblical creation of the world in seven days (remembering of course the day of rest at the end). Seven represents completion; as in the chakra work, each pupil completes him or herself in each of seven steps.

After seven years children lose their first teeth — Muladhara is associated with the teeth. After fourteen years, boys become men — here is the link with the Svadisthana Chakra. The period up to twenty-one is associated with growth and the centre of the body — the Manipura Chakra. Up to the 28th year growth is concentrated in broadening rather than growing tall — the Heart Chakra opens up the chest and the upper body. Between 28 and 35, people are at their greatest power: this is a function of the Throat Chakra, since you use your mind and communication skills to attain your greatest power.

From 35 onwards so much new experience is gained that a person is now able to develop into a fully mature individual.

This seven-year period corresponds with the astrological rhythm of Saturn. Every seven years Saturn is either in conjunction, opposition or square to the position it was in at the moment of birth — I am not sure whether this has any connection with the seven-year chakra cycle from Muladhara to Sahasrara, but I would imagine that this seven-year cycle would evolve to a new level each time it recurred. See if you can see any evidence for this in your own life.

Incidentally, the irrational number pi (π) can also be written as $^{22}/_7$. Thus the unlimited and the limited, thesquare and the circle, are connected by π. The circle of life.

"The life of the gods is mathematics" (Novalis).

1. The mantras are written in the way they are pronounced. In other books you may find them written as 'Lam', 'Vam', 'Ram', 'Yam' and 'Ham'. The pronunciation of the mantras is carefully described. You should make the syllable 'Lang' with a square mouth and a square tongue; 'Vang' like flowing water; 'Rang' with a triangular mouth, sounding like a burning fire; 'Yang' with your tongue free in your mouth (sounding like 'dschang'); and 'Hang' with oval lips, forcing the air out of your throat.

2. Where the different energy potentials of men and women are described, the negative energy symbol refers to potential energy and the positive symbol to kinetic energy. In the 'alchemical marriage' — the ritual sexual union — an energy exchange takes place between the chakras, thus activating the chakras of both the man and the woman. In Tantra you

will find lovemaking positions like the Sukhapadma Asana in which the partners activate all the chakras with the exception of the Ajna and Sahasrara Chakras. In Tantra this is known as 'closing the energy circle'.

3. The connection between the higher and the lower self is best understood in terms of gaining power from knowing what is truly meant to take place.

4. Crowley, Aleister *The Moonchild* Sphere, 1972.

5. The cardinal cross in astrology, and the Rajas in Indian philosophy, corresponds with the Muladhara and Manipura Chakras, giving us power and energy. The mutable cross in astrology, or Sattva, corresponds with the Visshuddha and Ajna Chakras, indicating the purpose of our lives (as does the third Norn — Skuld — in Germanic mythology). The fixed cross, or Tamas, corresponds with the Svadisthana and Anahata Chakras, which puts fate into our hands.

5

The Individual Chakras

Whether one envisages the chakras as round openings in the etheric body through which the physical body is connected by electromagnetic currents (a conventional concept that also needs to be seen metaphorically), or as a way of living and growing, the two should not be seen as contradictory. I see these two aspects of chakras as totally complementary.

In the text which follows I shall be taking the more conventional aspect of chakras into account whenever they seem to make sense, and help to clarify the ideas.

The seven chakras can also be thought of as having a vibration which resonates with each of the seven planets of classical astrology. Following the Rosicrucian tradition, we find the model presented by Table 4. The astrophysician Braunger bases his theories on the idea that we have today reached a stage of incomplete integration, which takes place in the higher frequencies of trans-Saturnine planetary vibrations. We should aim to let the chakras vibrate with the planets shown in the first column of Table 4. This involves the

Table 3
The Planetary Resonances of the Chakras

	Future	Today
SAHASRARA	♄	♅
AJNA	♅ ♆	⊕ ♆ ☿
VISHUDDHA	12th planet ♅	12th planet ♅
ANAHATA	Isis ♀	Isis ♀
MANIPURA	♃ ♂	♃ ♂
SVADISTHANA	☿ ☽	☿ ♆ ☽
MULADHARA	⊕	♀

transformation of the Sahasrara, Ajna, Svadisthana and Muladhara Chakras.[1]

If we think of the human being with its seven chakras as a complete field of vibrations, then the change of vibration in the upper two chakras will alter the whole energy field. This means that we must work on our grounding at the same time as we open up our spirit. The power to do this comes from the Heart Chakra, because it is here that the rising and falling energies (love and hate) meet each other. If we can harmonise the rising and falling energies, then we can open ourselves to the high frequency vibrations of the solar system. Thus we can reach complete harmony with the spirit of the times.

If we only tune into the lower frequencies of the lower chakras, we become rigid and stiff, but if we can tune into the frequencies of the higher chakras —

symbolised by the greater number of lotus leaves — then we not only allow our minds to become open and flexible, but with all seven chakras we will provide a perfect space for the resonance of all the vibrations of the solar system. Then we are perfectly grounded with our Base Chakra, and the Crown Chakra — with its Saturnine vibration — brings a clear understanding of the life we have lived up to the present. Tension (Mars) and relaxation (Jupiter) are in perfect balance at the Navel Chakra, and at the Heart Chakra the rising and falling energy streams are harmoniously combined (Isis and Venus). At the level of the Throat Chakra we are able to process neural and hormonal information without resistance (symbolised by the qualities of Uranus), and we are able to speed up our body rhythms, the expression of intuition (Uranus) translated into energy terms.

Developments in gestalt psychology in the 1920s and 30s showed that many of these ideas about energies fit in with field theory in psychological growth. The field model shows how the development of one chakra affects the overall development of the whole system. Thus you only need to heed fully the lessons of one chakra to be well on the way to opening all the chakras.

THE BASE CHAKRA[3]
MULADHARA

'Mulha' means 'bone marrow'.
Situated between the sacrum and the coccyx.

This chakra can be activated if you pause between breathing out and breathing in again. Activating the Base Chakra calms down the central nervous system and reduces the tension in your spine. But what does 'activating a chakra' mean?

Another way of activating the chakra is to concentrate on it, imagining it becoming warm and relaxed. Try breathing deeply into the chakra, then immediately after the outbreath concentrate on the feelings in that area of the body around the chakra.

The activation of a chakra cannot be done without first having worked on what you need to learn on the level of the particular chakra — this is a challenge that must be faced in day-to-day living.

You can also activate or stimulate a particular chakra by using particular asanas, mantras, and therapeutic techniques. We shall look at these in detail when we come to the exercises.

A chakra can be thought of as being activated if the principle of the chakra has been accepted as a lesson in everyday life — if the quality of the chakra can really be lived. This is also linked with the harmonising of the organ and glands associated with each particular chakra.

The lesson of the Muladhara Chakra is grounding. Too much yin means lack of grounding; too much yang means being too controlled.

Figure 6
The Spine seen from the Back
with the Locations of the Five Lower Chakras

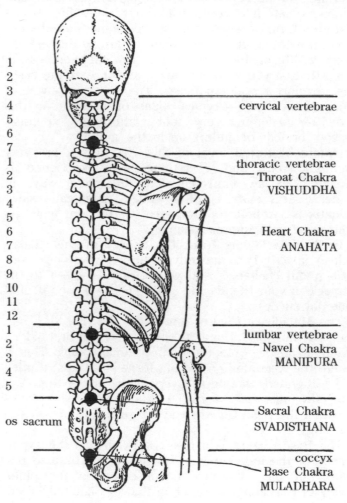

1
2
3
4   cervical vertebrae
5
6
7
1   thoracic vertebrae
2   Throat Chakra
3   VISHUDDHA
4
5
6   Heart Chakra
7   ANAHATA
8
9
10
11
12
1   lumbar vertebrae
2   Navel Chakra
3   MANIPURA
4
5

              Sacral Chakra
os sacrum   SVADISTHANA

              coccyx
              Base Chakra
              MULADHARA

J.T.C.—F

Physical mastery of the body is associated with the Base Chakra, the negative pole of the body. It is from this chakra that you find the energy to get up in the morning, the energy to start working. The Base Chakra connects you like roots with your daily life. In its distorted form — when there are resistances and blocks in the flow of energy — you tend to cling to the tasks of everyday life, unable to open up to joy and happiness. In this situation you work furiously, and in extreme cases can develop a real fanaticism. The creative power of work is blocked — typical signs of dis-ease on this level are becoming very poor without any apparent reason, or fear of ending up in the gutter.

On the distorted level of this chakra you are very impressionable, and everything you experience is reflected in an unifferentiated dreamlike way. In esoterics this state is often called 'Atlantean', since Atlantis is symbolic of that area of the soul which is connected with impressionability.

In its free-flowing form, the energy of this chakra helps you actively to master your life. You see your work as a joyful challenge, and you attract — often to the surprise of your friends and colleagues — a good deal of material success.

The Muladhara Chakra represents the first step into the material world. Using its energy you will find hidden within it all the potential of the human being. This is where the Kundalini — the life force — sleeps, waiting to be liberated, waiting to give you the power to go out into the material world. I find many similarities between the Base Chakra and the principle of Aries in astrology.

The Base Chakra is a reservoir where all the experiences of the individual are stored, and it is also one aspect of the 'collective unconscious' in the philosophy of Carl Jung, or of 'id' in that of Sigmund Freud.

THE SACRAL CHAKRA
SVADISTHANA

Situated between the fifth lumbar vertebra and the os sacrum.

This energy can be activated using the same breathing technique as for activating the Base Chakra — pausing briefly after the outbreath to let the energy move down the spine.

The activation of this chakra regulates and harmonises the fluids in the human body, thus affecting the urogenital system, and easing arthritis and diseases of the blood. Women's disorders can also be relieved by the activation of the Sacral Chakra, or perhaps it is more correct to say that activation of this chakra is a powerful preventative against women's disorders. The activation of this chakra also helps the enjoyment of a satisfying sexual life.

The lesson of the Sacral Chakra is creativity.

Too much yin results in sexual difficulties like impotency and frigidity, following from a weakening of the lower body. Too much yang results in sexual overactivity: nymphomania and the Don Juan syndrome — though these concepts arise largely from a moralistic viewpoint rather than a psychological one.

With the Svadisthana Chakra we reach the level of giving and receiving. On the physical level this is represented by the digestive system; on the emotional level by the ability to surrender, to give and receive; and on the intellectual level by the ability to store information and integrate knowledge. The relevant question here is: Am I able to live what I know? In short, this chakra involves giving and receiving at all levels.

In the distorted form there is a disharmony of giving
and receiving, disturbing the natural flow of energy. This
distortion can lead to obesity in people whose taking
has outgrown their capacity for giving — they cannot
give away enough of what they cannot digest. The
opposite syndrome is anorexia nervosa. Here also we
find people — and which of us does not recognise ourself
in this? — who use sexual encounter as a way of getting
attention. Here is a desire to be acknowledged, coming
from a deep fear of never being able to give enough; the
erotic-narcissistic game of flirting.

On the free-flowing level we find the people who can
let go, who can become fully involved in projects in
which they can behave originally and creatively with
other people. They can combine an intellectual analysis
of the world with their desires and emotions. You are
able to let yourself in, knowing that you are lovable just
the way you are. You are able to work creatively with
other people, especially when their perspective differs
from your own — you complement each other well. This
is the foundation of all creativity: combining differing
lifestyles, meanings and expressions, seeing all these
things reflected in yourself, and so learning to become a
whole and complete human being.

Try meditating on these lines of Heraclitus:

"Opposites always complement each other.
The loveliest harmonies arise from differences."

The lessons of this chakra should always be seen from
the point of view of opposites.

Jung saw this energy centre as reflecting an ancient
level of consciousness, when human beings lived like fish
in the ocean of the unconscious.[3] At that time, when
there was no ego-consciousness to interrupt the
natural flow, there was never any problem in giving and
receiving.

THE NAVEL CHAKRA
MANIPURA

Also called the Hara or Solar Plexus Chakra.
Situated between the twelfth thoracic vertebra and
the first lumbar vertebra.

This chakra can be activated by concentrating on the
chakra and breathing into it without taking any break
between inbreath and outbreath, or between outbreath
and inbreath, breathing deeply and regularly through
the nose (a common practice in yoga).

The activation of this chakra (as the shamans have
discovered) has a positive effect on all illnesses and
disturbances which have their roots in internalised
aggression, including cancer and other tumours. It also
has a healing effect on diseases of the stomach, which
are often connected with anger.

This level is generally to do with power, will, ambition,
wants and desires.

The lesson of this chakra is dealing with power.

Too much yin results in powerlessness; too much yang
in aggression and greed.

Just as when you learned to survive on the material
level when you reached the Muladhara Chakra, so you
met the 'other' at the level of the Svadisthana and
shared with them, and now you reach the centre of the
body, your point of gravity. Here you meet daily life with
all its challenges and problems, and you meet it with
your will and your power. There is no way of avoiding the
battle, and nobody will come out of it without really
learning to fight.

But there are many ways of fighting. In the distorted
form you can easily fall back into the old way in which

you fight 'an eye for an eye and a tooth for a tooth'. It
is only from bitter experience that you learn that it is
the inflexible and rigid who always lose.

Seen from the point of view of the alchemists, this is
the level at which material and its energies are transformed into mind and higher vibrational forms. Here,
therefore, you will find the organs of stomach, liver and
gall bladder.

In everyday life you have to purify your will and your
desires. In a way you 'raise' them to another level by
investing them with social responsibility. This is the
chakra of the shamans, since its aim is to look after
social relationships. It is also associated with communication with the world of spirits — with dark archaic
powers.

The alchemical parallel with this chakra is called Sol
Niger (black sun) or Caput Corvi (raven's head), the
principle idea of Saturn.

This suggests the importance of recognising your own
dark side, and it is in conflict situations that you can
experience this best. The first step in dealing with your
dark side is to see it clearly, the second step to accept
it — fighting against it will only make it more rigid. The
third step lies in transforming your dark side into
'positive battle'.

For me, positive battle has to do with an acceptance
of your own anger, and also with deep insight into social
responsibility. The positive fighter does not fight to
destroy the other person, though they are not afraid to
show their anger as an important part of the whole
person, all the time aware that the anger is their own
responsibility. The positive fighter does not create
distance by projecting the anger on to other people; if
you are a positive fighter you are fully aware that the
anger is only to do with yourself. By showing your anger
clearly from this perspective, you are able to express

something which is deeply felt, and communicate part of that self to your social group or community, without needing to withdraw.

The negative aggression which seeks to destroy others is thus transformed into a positive initiative which helps people to understand themselves, making it clear that anger is part of being human but without hiding it. In the end, dealing in this way with the 'dark side' means that it will no longer be dark.

Using free-flowing energy on this level allows you to use your intuition in the face of apparent danger. Put another way, you find the guardian angel in yourself.

If you are not able to deal with these challenges within yourself, dealing with your dark side and the necessary social limitations upon it, you will be in danger of developing neuroses, which are the breeding ground of black magic. To me black magic means using your power to manipulate other people with your selfish actions.

In the end every individual human being has to decide how to deal with this level, between earth and heaven. Will you travel the path of the heart and try to raise your energies to the higher levels, or will you go on the path of materialism and reason, which may mean losing contact with the soul?

We live constantly with this contradiction, and it is a brave person who can aim for both at the same time. In our deterministic and materialistic culture, however, the first step of integrating both paths is usually to develop your spirit as part of the path towards heaven.

It is within the apparent contradiction that the personality, with its responsibilities, is formed. If we have decided upon the path of light (as Alice Bailey and Olga von Ungern-Sternberg call it), we come at this level — the Manipura Chakra — to an inner initiation.

THE HEART CHAKRA
ANAHATA

This is the central chakra, and consistent with Goethe's colour theory, in which green is at the centre of the colour circle, I connect it with the colour green. It is situated between the fourth and fifth thoracic vertebrae.

This chakra can be enhanced using the same breathing technique as for the Manipura Chakra, but you should concentrate on your heartbeat without attempting to change it. You might try the autogenic (self-hypnosis) technique of saying to yourself: 'My heart beats quietly and regularly.'

The activation of this chakra heals the heart and stabilises the blood circulation.

Having experienced our 'dark side' in the struggle of life, with the Anahata Chakra you now reach the level of peace and harmony. You can now be a constructive social being (as in the Greek ideal of the Zoon Politikon), discovering the warmth of your heart as a creative force in social settings. The social responsibility learnt at the last step can now be developed into real social awareness.

The lesson of the Anahata Chakra is social awareness, love and openness.

Too much yin leads to insensitivity; too much yang to oversensitivity.

With the Heart Chakra you can develop the theme of meeting with 'the other' more fully, a theme we first explored with the Sacral Chakra. This time, however, we have moved on from sexual encounter and intimate meetings, to a wider group consciousness. The lesson of this chakra might be expanded as 'the integration of the self into larger social groups'.

In the distorted form of the Anahata Chakra, even though you may have learnt the right way of fighting at the Manipura level, you may still remain overly cool and intellectually distanced in conflicts. In psychoanalysis this is called 'defence by rationalisation'.

This is a particular problem for people with water signs, who often react very calmly when offended or insulted in contradiction to their true deep feelings. Supressing your feelings by smoking is a very common reaction at this level, and this often indicates a reluctance to feel your real feelings, similar to what in bioenergetics is known as the 'breast block'.

In its free-flowing form, we find in this chakra the positive qualities of the astrological concept of Leo: being able to serve a wider group through your talents for organisation, social skills and diplomacy. You are able to integrate and adapt yourself without losing your identity in the process.

Like the Hanged Man in the Tarot, we find many powerful and gifted people at this level who are able to see and combine many different perspectives at the same time.

THE THROAT CHAKRA
VISHUDDHA

Situated between the seventh cervical vertebra and the first thoracic vertebra.

This chakra can be stimulated by pausing after the inbreath. In this way the energies can be encouraged to rise. The pause should never be held longer than is

comfortable. Taking a short pause after the inbreath
allows the energies to rise (a pause taken after the
outbreath allows them to fall) — especially if you
push the inhaled air up into your thorax during the
pause.

It seems to me that the Vishuddha Chakra is the
easiest to stimulate by breathing. By activating this
chakra the quality of your voice will become fuller,
clearer and deeper. Activating the Throat Chakra will
help to alleviate hoarseness, and the stimulation of the
Throat Chakra is part of the training of professional
singers. Problems with the functioning of the thyroid
gland — which are difficult to treat any other way —
can be improved by working on the Throat Chakra, as
can depressive tendencies in the hormonal system.

What is the principle of the Throat Chakra? First, it
can help us to cleanse the lower chakras.

This is where you very consciously connect the
thoughts and feelings from your path so far, reflecting
clearly on what you have learned. You start to understand your path, and can see it as a whole. This is why
language and communication are so important at this
level — talking with other people, reading the books
which help you to clarify and understand your life up to
now. You are able to see the spiritual implications of
your chosen path, able to see the consequences of the
decisions you have made during difficult situations.

Until you have undertaken this 'cleansing', this
integration, it is difficult to claim your own history, to
turn inwardly in a truly positive way.

It is at this level that thinking and feeling are
connected most intimately, forming the foundation
upon which you make the next two steps, the steps up
to the level of the thousandfold lotus where you can act
from your intuition at every level — where the principle
of Uranus becomes a reality.

But back to the Throat Chakra — we cannot miss out important steps or take short cuts. The key here is assimiliation. Everything you have so far learned in your life must be looked at from the deep and spiritual point of view, but you must also find a way of communicating these insights with the outside world. The aim is clear communication of your life's experiences. This is where your education for the spiritual level begins.

But what does 'spiritual' mean?

At this level, dreamwork can be very useful, because the ego in your dreams precisely reflects the actions, sorrows and joys of your conscious ego. In dreamwork these subconscious insights can be made conscious, and thereby translated into the outside world as creative and formative action. This process can be assisted by using the Bach flower remedies Cerato and Scleranthus.

The lesson of the Vishuddha Chakra is communication and assimilation. Too much yin creates problems in communication and an inability to express yourself clearly. Too much yang results in a tendency to dominate any form of communication.

The five chakras we have looked at so far, together with their qualities, can be thought of as points on the spine (see Figure 6). They can be set free by touching, breathing, concentration, visualisation, and working with the problems associated with them.

These five energy points can also be thought of as the points of a pentagram. In the pentagram, all five energies have to be in balance, otherwise unbalancing influences can affect the person concerned.[4] In chakra work this means that we need to develop all five chakras and their qualities in harmony with each other to enable us to reach the spiritual qualities of the Ajna and Sahasrara Chakras.

If these five chakras and the qualities associated with them are lived in harmony, that individual human being will have developed a whole and satisfying way of life. According to Ungern-Sternberg, the pentagram is a powerful symbol, representing an inner balance reflected in action in the world. This is just another way of expressing the aim of chakra work, which is responsible social action based on the integration of inner experience.

"When the five powers are in harmony, the devil can never intrude. We shall never fall into the Faustian trap; never be tempted to remain anonymous and irresponsible."

Figure 7
The Lower Five Chakras as a Pentagram

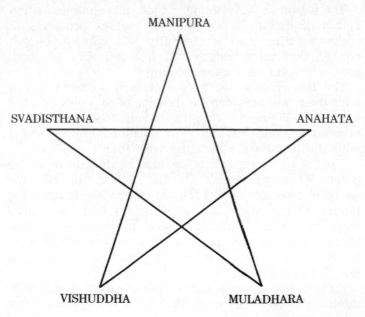

The last two chakras can be thought of as being situated in the skull.

THE THIRD EYE
AJNA

In classical yoga teachings, the Ajna Chakra is sometimes thought of as an inner energy centre under the Sahasrara Chakra.
It is situated at the meeting of two energy lines, one of which joins the ear cavities, the other passing from the base of your nose to the back of your head.

Like the Vishuddha Chakra, the Ajna Chakra can be stimulated by pausing after the inbreath. The activation of this chakra has physiological effects, and can be a powerful way of overcoming anxiety. In the end, all tension is rooted in fear: deep breathing into this chakra while repeating the 'aum' mantra can dissolve fear, grief and nightmares, and if done frequently it can deal with all stress. This will only happen, however, if you work regularly with this chakra, and try to live your life in accordance with its principles. If you can move beyond your fears and really let go, then you will reach a new level of concentration, and notice a qualitative change in your meditation.

If you are able to watch your thoughts and feelings during meditation without being concerned about them, you will now be ready to use this practised emptiness to focus your thoughtforms like a laser beam on any point in the universe. Wherever you are you will be able to understand everything about the world, and begin to see the universe as a huge hologram, in which everything is reflected in everything else.

You will be able to send love, light and healing energy to everyone you love, and know that although it may sometimes be hard to believe, these energies really will be received.

The lesson of the Ajna Chakra is imagination and concentration. When the yin and yang are unbalanced, you may suffer from headaches and problems with your concentration.

At this level we take our powers of positive thinking and creative visualisation out into the world. In the final analysis, positive thinking and constructive visualisation are not possible until you have reached this level, because only now will you know what you want for the true welfare of yourself and of others. By now you should know that working with your dark side helps it to become lighter and lighter, and you should have no problem with your concentration. Though I may be naive in my belief, I am certain that we only reach this level of power when we know how to handle it correctly and ethically. Yet there is misuse of this power, though we must always ask ourselves whether such misuse might not in the end serve some larger goal. I find this hard to believe when I think for instance of Adolf Hitler, but these are delicate questions, and I am not wise enough to answer them.

When are you mature enough to handle this amount of power?

What power do you truly have?

How did you reach the level when you were able to deal with it correctly and ethically?

Attitudes towards ethical responsibility are a real area of conflict within spirituality. There is an enormous range of opinion, varying from the enlightened to the devilishly destructive — one only has to think of

Aleister Crowley and Gurdjieff to see the different ways that power can be used. In the *Mabinogion* the evil sorceress utters the words of power, and in the process destroys herself.

One of the main things to be developed at this level is the so-called 'intelligence of the heart'. Using your love, your intelligence and your intuition together, you can use your imagination actively to help build a new world.

In the distorted form of the energy of this chakra you cease to believe in anything, often sinking into a deep and cynical nihilism, which reflects your inability to believe in important ideas and great visions. And you are to blame, no one else. You believe that the guilt is not yours, unable to see that you have attracted the situation and the people in it.

Perhaps this is the place to say that I do not believe that it is always necessary to work with the chakras in their 'correct order'. This is only an ideal model. More usually you will find yourself working on several levels at the same time, though at different levels of consciousness.

You may find that you are able to free your upper chakras to a large extent, but still have problems with being grounded in everyday life. Ideally, all the chakras should be stimulated so they are in balance with each other, but the complete freeing of the upper chakras can only be based on free-flowing energy in the lower chakras, because of their synergistic character. If you cannot satisfy your basic needs, you will always have problems when it comes to working on the spiritual levels.

THE CROWN CHAKRA
SAHASRARA

Also called 'the thousandfold lotus'. Because this
chakra is largely beyond language and beyond our
space-time continuum, there is little that can be said
about it.
It is situated at the acupuncture point called Tou Mo*,
in the middle of the crown of the skull at the meeting
point of the fontanelles.

This chakra is concerned with the many aspects of
cosmic programming which are higher than our
individual self, and which are beyond our powers of
comprehension. Here the lower and higher selves are
fused, and there is absolute trust. There is no more
unconscious, and no possibility of distortion.
    In everyday life you will want what happens anyway;
action and understanding become one. In the Tantra it
is said that the inner core of Sahasrara consists of three
parts: Bindu[5], Bija[6] and Nada[7]. This is where Shiva
(semen) and Shakti (menstrual blood) combine as Shiva-
Shakti in the 'alchemical marriage', the fusion of the
higher and lower selves.
    Here I will allow myself a few thoughts about
enlightenment. For me there can be no enlightenment
on earth, in the sense that all tensions can be overcome.

---

* This point is also sometimes called Paihui or Baihui; it
means 'the meeting point of the hundred ways', because this
is where all the yang meridians meet. There is a parallel
between this point and Jung's archetype of the horned god,
since both symbolise the energy patterns of the open
Sahasrara Chakra (see Patricia Garfield, *The Way of the
Dream Mandala*, New York, 1979, pp.192-206).

I find the idea of being totally relaxed in the here and now rather naive and dangerous. The world is full of life because it contains tensions, joys and sorrows — all these are essential parts of life. What I do believe is that these can all be dealt with creatively at the level of the Sahasrara Chakra.

For me the vision of total harmony and relaxation in the here and now seems dead — life is a challenge because of its tensions; this is what makes life worthwhile.

1. Field theory, as it has been developed in gestalt therapy by analogy with the new physics, is very similar to a holographic view of the universe. In each field every vibrational pattern reflects the structure of the whole field.

2. For the connections between the chakras and the elements, see Table 2.

3. Jung, C.G. *The Tree of Philosophy* Routledge.

4. See the 'Easter Walk' scene in Goethe's *Faust.*

5. Bindu — the power and energy of the Shiva principle, symbolised by the colour white, and by the moon. It represents the male semen, and can be freely translated as 'will'.

6. Bija — the power and energy of the Shakti principle, symbolised by the colour red, and by fire. It represents menstrual blood, and can be freely translated as 'action'.

7. Nada — the fusion of Shiva and Shakti, symbolised by red and white, and by the sun. It can be translated freely as 'understanding' or 'sound'.

The figure on the next page shows the connection between the three principles:

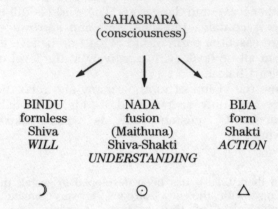

6
Deciding Which Chakra to Work on First

You may find it difficult to know which of your chakras you want to start working on, where it is that there may be too little or too much energy. One way of finding this out is to try the muscle testing technique used by practitioners of homoeopathy and the Bach flower remedies.

To do this in a very simple way, you will need a friend to help you. Stand up and stretch your right arm out straight ahead of you, palm down; your left hand (which is receiving energy) should be placed first at the Sahasrara Chakra, then at each of the other chakras down through the body. As you touch each chakra, your friend should put their hand on and above your forearm — they should say 'Now try to resist' as they push gently downwards on your forearm, and you should gently try to resist the pressure. This is done for each of the seven chakras.

If the resistance is strong, then that chakra has a lot of energy, and if the resistance is weak that particular chakra is low in energy. You are receiving this energy

with your left hand, which is immediately reflected in
the rest of the body, including your right arm — there is
never too much energy in one part of the body without
there being too little in another. If the muscle test
indicates that the resistance of all seven chakras is
much the same, this suggests that the chakras are in
harmony.

This is only one of several muscle tests that can be
used. The 'Touch for Health' technique uses many of
these muscle tests, and you might like to read John
Thie's *Touch for Health*[1] for more ideas. All muscle
tests are basically the same, but I have found that this
one is particularly good at differentiating between the
energy levels of the different chakras.

Another easy muscle test you can use to explore the
energy patterns of your chakras is one which uses the
fingers. Touch the tip of your right little finger with the
tip of your right thumb, holding your left hand on the
chakra you are testing. Now ask your friend to pull the
finger and thumb apart, checking the resistance as you
move your left hand down through the chakras. I often
use this test because it can be done so quickly, and
because the muscles of the right hand do not tire as
easily as your arm muscles in the previous test.

Why not try the thumb-and-finger test now (if you
can find someone to help you), and see if you can relate
the results to your everyday life?

Even if you choose not to work on the weakest
chakra first, it is important to work on the weak
chakras as well as the one you do choose. If there is a
considerable imbalance between the chakras, it is a
good idea to use on a regular basis some exercises that
stimulate all the chakras. These exercises will be found
in the last chapter but one.

1. Thie, John and Mary Marks *Touch for Health* Santa
Monica, 1973.

7
Red Tantra
A Digression

I want to mention briefly that the chakras are always stimulated during sexual union with another person; even though it is unconscious, love-making activates the chakras, and it is important to be aware the links between the chakras and the senses.

On the level of the Muladhara Chakra the sense of smell is important — the smell of the genitals as well as the sweet smell of the skin. At the level of the Svadisthana Chakra you taste the saltiness of the skin and the discharge of the genitals. At the Manipura level it is important to see the naked bodies — this can be a powerful meditation. At the Anahata level, touching and feeling are important. On the Vishuddha level, you tune into all the sounds of your partner, from the beating of their heart to their cries of passion.

The development of each of these senses can be used as a way of nurturing your relationship with your partner.

A good exercise at the level of the Manipura Chakra is to meditate on the naked body of your partner. We have all surely done this at one time or another, but now we can learn to enjoy the sight of their naked body with new and concentrated awareness.

Sit in a meditative position in front of your partner, so that you can see each other's genitals clearly. Now breathe deeply and regularly without pausing, concentrating the breath into the genitals. Without moving, concentrate your eyes on your partner's gentals for at least a quarter of an hour. Now close your eyes and visualise in detail what you have seen, drawing it into yourself. You may now decide whether or not you want to make love.

Sexual arousal can be built up through all the chakras, from the feet (Muladhara), to the hands (Svadisthana) and the anus (Manipura), then slowly into the vagina and clitoris or the penis. Hold back the ecstasy as long as possible, building up the tension in these chakras. If you concentrate on the order of the chakras from the feet to the hands to the anus to the genitals, you will be able to feel the rising current of excitement quite clearly.

Because women and men have opposite energy charges in the different chakras, an intensive current of energy can be built up during love-making. In its culmination (and without any conscious effort), the two upper chakras will be activated.

In certain Asanas (for example the Sukhapadma and the Yoni Asana), it is very important that the partners touch each other's chakras, with the exception of the Sahasrara Chakra.

The Sahasrara Chakra is a symbol of the fusion of Shiva and Shakti, and has a neutral charge in both men and women[1]; at this level you cannot help to liberate each other. Sahasrara reflects the individual experience of ecstasy, whereas the other chakras reflect the aspect of sharing. If you are interested in reading more about this path, look at the asanas, exercises and meditations in John Mumford's book *Sexual Occultism*[2].

It is important to be aware that in Tibetan Buddhism (Vayrayana and Tantrayana), Tantra has little to do with sexual practice. The images of sexual union (known as Yab-Yum, the father and mother aspects of Buddha) symbolise the fusion of wisdom (the mother) and method (the father). The purpose of these images is to symbolise the transformation of sexuality into spirit.

The common picture of Tantra in the West subverts Buddhist Tantra into its exact opposite. When I talk about 'Red Tantra' (as opposed to Black and White Tantra), I am referring to the ancient sexual magical rites of Hinduism, in which enlightenment is to be found in women's genitalia. Particularly in our patriarchal society, it is important to acknowledge that the full and active sexual arousal of a woman is a powerful means of self-expression — the body never lies. This kind of sexuality, however, must be preceded by the development of a certain level of awareness.

I believe that we in the West are capable of recognising sexual powers in an aware way, and that given a heightened level of awareness we can use these powers wisely when we come together in love. As in the chakra work, whether we free ourselves or limit ourselves is a question of consciousness, and this is particularly important when it comes to sexuality.

Chakra work encourages us to see sexuality as part of the whole human being, not just as an isolated phenomenon which sometimes uses all our energies. I can understand those Theosophists and Anthroposophists who warn against working with the sexual chakra. In a world that insists on working everything out analytically, working with our sexuality can easily attract too much attention, detracting from the belief that the human being is a whole being, spiritual as well as sexual.

1. For the energy charges of the chakras of women and men, see Table 2.

2. Mumford, John *Sexual Occultism* U.S.A., 1975. See also Culling, Louis T. *The Complete Magic Curriculum of the Secret Order G.B.G.* Llewellyn, U.S.A., 1970. It is probably best for you and your partner to develop exercises of your own. Most of the books you will find on the market which include sections on Tantra, Red Tantra or Sexual Magic are complete nonsense.

8
The Exercises

PHYSICAL EXERCISES
ASANAS

These exercises are a combination of classical yoga
asanas, bioenergetic exercises, Gurdjieff movements,
and direct communication with your body.

I have combined the activation of certain acupuncture points with the yoga asanas in order to become
aware in a very immediate way of the currents of energy
flowing through the body. Over the years, however, I
have stopped looking for specific acupuncture points —
I always had problems remembering exactly where they
were. But then I noticed that my hands would find the
places that needed to be massaged; now I trust the
intuition of my hands, and I don't think it matters very
much whether I am working exactly on a particular
acupuncture point. Tuning into your body is far more
important than learning the fine detail of a particular
system. Emphasis on the system detracts from the all-
important listening to your body.

Perhaps we can see working with intuition as a female way, and working with a system as a male way. As a man, it seems very important to me to develop this intuition in a way that is rarely practised in our society; maybe women need to develop their systematic side.

All these body exercises involve stretching the muscles. This stretching should never be forced. If it hurts you or is very uncomfortable it will simply be building up more tension than it is relieving. If it does hurt it shows that you are stretching too much or in the wrong way, and you should immediately stop doing that particular exercise.

Never push or rock your body while you stretch, because this can easily cause you to overdo the stretching. Move slowly into a stretched position, keeping your breathing deep and regular. If you cannot maintain this pattern of breathing — especially if you have to hold your breath or are reduced to gasping — you are using your will too much, and are in danger of hurting yourself. Maintaining deep and regular breathing will allow you to relax deeply into the position.

To begin with you should maintain these body positions for no more than a minute; you can gradually increase this to about five minutes.

BREATHING
PRANAYAMA

In yoga and chakra work there are two different kinds of breathing; concentrated and conscious breathing, and held breath. According to the yoga literature, controlled pauses in breathing can lead to experiencing psi phenomena; in my opinion it is not as easy as that. The literature also suggests that breathing affects the

Kundalini. I cannot agree that deep breathing, or indeed any form of breathing, can *alone* affect the Kundalini or help you to reach higher consciousness. For breathing to be effective within yoga and chakra work, it must be seen as part of a holistic approach which also involves bodywork, and mental and emotional development.

I will not go into techniques for holding the breath here, since if they are not used very carefully and gently they can easily damage your health. In my chakra work I only use concentrated breathing without holding the breath for very long. In Tibetan Buddhism this concentrated breathing is called 'riding the horse of the breath': the idea is that after a while the breathing will be in control of itself, and you will feel as though you are 'being breathed'.

Breathing into the chest and breathing into the stomach both have their advantages and disadvantages. Breathing into your stomach can quieten your thoughts and help you to be perfectly grounded; breathing into the chest can help you to raise your energies. Integrated yoga breathing breathes into the stomach and the chest at the same time.

Deep and regular breathing provides a way of relaxing, and you can direct your breathing to those parts of the body where you are experiencing resistance and tension. When the tension has been dissolved, you can stop breathing into the area and, lying on your back, relax by breathing in and out without pausing, as in rebirthing. The tense places will probably now start to tremble, thus releasing the blocked energies.

It is always important to breathe naturally, in your own rhythm, not forcing yourself into a certain pattern. Even if you are breathing without pausing (as I have described above), do not force yourself into hyperventilating. If for some reason you need to hyperventilate, your body will naturally lead you to it.

Your energy level is largely dependent on your
breathing, and ultimately on the way you live your
whole life.[1] If in the following exercises you just follow
your natural pattern of breathing, you will find as you
work on your chakras that your breathing will change,
almost unconsciously.

The relation between inhaling and exhaling reflects
how you receive and give, how you hold back and let go.

Have you ever noticed that anger makes it very hard
to breathe properly?

Sit down with your spine straight, close your eyes,
and let the back of your hands rest on your knees.
Now touch the tip of each thumb to the tip of the
index finger on each hand and stretch the other
fingers (the Inana Mudra). Sit for about five minutes,
and breathe in your natural rhythm, watching your
breathing all the time but without changing it or
trying to control it. Where do you feel resistance?
What are your feelings?

Your index finger symbolises your personal soul, your
thumb the universal soul — think about the importance
of the opposing thumb in the evolution of human beings.
With the flow of your breathing you are completing the
cycle of energy exchange between the individual and the
universal soul.

As you breathe, watch the feelings arise which are
normally supressed. Look at those feelings.

Integrated yoga breathing uses the stomach, the
chest and the collarbones, but do not worry about this
too much at the beginning. The most important thing is
to find your own pattern of breathing — this is what
brings you into harmony, and balances the acid and
alkali in your body.

THE MIND

The only authentic source of yoga, the *Yoga Sutra* of
Patanjali, says:
'*Yoga chitta vritti niroddah*'
(Yoga dissolves what hums in our heads)
To me this does not mean that you have to stop
thinking. Thought and intellect are both parts of the
whole, and reflect your inner divinity just as much as
feeling or any other aspect. I believe this sentence of
Patanjali is asking us to take our thinking more seriously, to become more aware of it, so that we can stop
it when we do not need it. It is when your thoughts are
uncontrolled that your head starts to hum, just like the
muzak in a supermarket. You need to work towards
being conscious of your thoughts, having your attention
focused, seeing things more impersonally — in short,
not getting attached. It is when we see reality exactly
as it is that tensions between body, mind and spirit
dissolve.

All the following exercises contain elements of
meditation, affirmation and visualisation.

Meditation involves letting go of the intellect
(remember what I said earlier about the principle of
Mercury). During your meditation, look at whatever
comes up. Look at it without hanging on to it and
without identifying with it. Meditating in this way
gives you the opportunity to use the light of your
insight to look at your shadow. What is your dark side?

Your shadow is everything in yourself that you find
hard to accept, and which you therefore project away
from yourself. Your shadow side is bound to come up
during meditation. Look at it and accept it.

You can use symbols or themes in your meditation.

We shall use this type of meditation when we come to the different chakras. You will make all sorts of associations with these themes and symbols — do not reject anything that comes up for you.

It is not particularly important to understand everything. In the Tarot meditations, for example, it is not important to understand the cabalistic implications of the cards — in fact knowing too much about the cards probably means that you end up knowing less about yourself. Just see what arises as you meditate on these archetypal pictures. It isn't a question of understanding the cards; it is about understanding yourself!

The three classical techniques of meditation in the chakra work are:

1. Concentration on the Ajna Chakra with your eyes closed, going with the flow of energy.
2. Staring at the tip of your nose with half-closed eyes (a sort of blinking), following the rhythm of your breathing.
3. Staring at one point with your eyes open.

You should at least try each of these techniques. From a physiological point of view, these meditations activate your hypothalamus and help to harmonise your hormone system.

At the end of the exercises associated with each individual chakra you will find affirmations. The use of affirmations comes from Tantric Buddhism[2], and affirmations work by internalising a positive message that you tell yourself.

In their books, the two friends Marcus Allen and Shakti Gawain[3] have set out the basic rules governing the way that affirmations work.

An affirmation says that something is going to be just how you want it to be.

An affirmation is always simply and positively worded.

It can be said out loud, or silently during meditation. I find that affirmations work best when I write them down.

An affirmation should have an emotional significance for you.

Working with affirmations is a sort of self-programming technique. It is based on the idea that everything must be created at the level of mind before it can manifest in the world. This is also the basic idea behind Tantra, whatever the particular form it takes.

By using meditation and affirmation in your yoga and chakra work you can use your intellect creatively, and overcome your limitations and inflexibility.

THERAPY

Here I want to mention a technique I often use in conjunction with my chakra work. Called Jin Shin Jyutzu, it is based on twenty-six points of the body which all have a spiritual significance. When you treat yourself or another person, you always connect two of these points with your right and left hands in a special order. Because the right hand has a positive energy charge (yang, giving) and the left a negative one (yin, receiving), you create a flow of energy between each pair of points which can help subtle problems to emerge in a very dreamlike way, and allow them to be dissolved.

Now that I have been working with this technique for some time I do not stick rigidly with the twenty-six points, and concentrate my work on the seven chakras and the tip of the nose (where the Ida and Pingala currents meet). In its notion of the 'small middle line', classical Jin Shin Jyutzu also tends to work with the chakras.

'I stand firmly within life, which I create lovingly and imaginatively.'

In the following exercises I shall suggest which points to touch, but you may well find that others are more useful for you. There are no limits to your creativity.

I also think of the use of mantras as a therapeutic aspect of chakra work, since there are many acupuncture points in the mouth which are stimulated when you pronounce the mantras in a certain order. If you repeat a particular mantra, you are stimulating specific acupuncture points, which has exactly the same effect as acupuncture or acupressure.

In classical chakra work, you always start by saying three times the mantra 'Ong Namo Guru Dev Namo' (this is how it is pronounced).

PREPARING FOR THE EXERCISES

I always start my preparations by tidying up my room. If my physical surroundings are tidy, then I feel I am also tidying up myself. Then I wash and change into some comfortable clothes. I always make sure that I shall not be disturbed for at least an hour. I do my chakra work in complete silence, which is easy for someone who lives in the country. When I lead workshops in cities I use soft meditative music — usually classical music — to cover the traffic noise.

I work alternately in the mornings and evenings, since both have their advantages and disadvantages. In the morning the body is relatively stiff but the head is quite empty; I feel quieter and more relaxed, and the chakra work gives me energy and power for the rest of the day. In the evening I can move more easily, but I have less concentration. On the other hand I like to end a working day with the exercises.

If I do the exercises in the evening, as a final meditation exercise I go back over the whole day, working backwards through everything that has happened. I look at my feelings and my moods, my successes and failures.

There are also very good reasons for doing your yoga at the same time every day. It can be helpful to condition yourself to expect 'yoga time' at the same time each day, a discipline that comes easily and is reinforced by the yoga itself. This discipline will help you to achieve a higher level of relaxation and concentration, and doing your yoga at the same time each day provides a useful structure for the rest of your life.

The Tibetans say you should always do your chakra work in the same place, too, since this brings discipline to the particular place as well as to you.

Pranayama Yoga suggests that yoga should always be done in the same lotus or half lotus position.

I never work with more than one chakra at each session, and I would recommend this way of working. It is impossible to go as deeply into more than one chakra as you can when you concentrate just on one.

Women should not try to do the asanas in the first month after giving birth. During menstruation it is wise not to do the asanas which stretch your body with the feet upwards, and you should not breath intensely into your stomach.

Since we are not attempting to raise the Kundalini, it is not necessary to practise sexual abstinence.

SOME FINAL TIPS

Here are a few thoughts which might help you:
    It helps if you are just slightly hungry.

J.T.C.—H

Face towards the east or towards the light (whether it be a window or a candle). Always move first to the right, since this is the direction of movement of the solar system. Never force anything.

You might like to pause here and write down the things that are important to you. Remember that this is constantly changing.

Enjoy yourself!

I know I have spent a long time explaining what chakra work is all about, but I believe that there is no better way for the student of the chakras to remain on the right path than to understand clearly the aims and principles of the chakra exercises.

1. Selby, John *Responsive Breathing* U.S.A., 1984.

2. Allen, Marcus *Tantra For the West* Whatever, U.S.A., 1981.

3. Gawain, Shakti *Creative Visualization* Whatever, U.S.A., 1978.

9
Exercises for
the Seven Chakras

THE BASE CHAKRA
MULADHARA

I start with a meditation on Tarot card number III, The Empress.

After meditating, I always do some grounding exercises. One very powerful method of grounding is a jumping exercise.

Sit comfortably on the floor, with the top of your feet and the front of your shins touching the floor and your heels uppermost (see Photo 1). Concentrate on a point about a foot in front of you — this is the point to which you will be jumping. Imagine that you will very soon jump to this point and land there safely. With your feet firmly on the ground, and feeling the ground supporting you, move slowly into a squatting position (Photo 2), then stand up. When you are clear within yourself about what you are doing and the order of doing it, jump to this point.

The energy to jump in this meditation comes from the Muladhara Chakra. This grounding exercise has more to do with trust than with strength — the faith that you will land safely, with the soles of both feet on the floor. This is an excellent way of overcoming the fears and blocks that will arise while you prepare for the exercise. Watch your arms, for example: do they trust your body, or is there a tendency for them to want to support it?

It is quite normal not to be able to master this exercise immediately. After the exercise, come up from the squatting position and stand up straight with your eyes closed, breathing deeply and regularly into your Muladhara Chakra. Imagine that you have roots that go deep into the ground; feel the energies flow from the Muladhara Chakra down to the centre of the earth and back again.

For the next exercise, sit on the floor with your legs stretched straight out in front of you. Try to keep your spine straight. You can control the straightness of your spine more easily if you have a mirror that you can put on the floor to one side of you. If you use this method for a while, you will soon come to know what having a straight spine feels like. Holding your right leg straight, move your left leg backwards by bending it at the knee. While breathing out, bend your body slowly down towards the straight leg, and touch your right foot with your hands. Hold your foot or leg (wherever is comfortable to reach) for about a minute, then loose your hands slowly and return to sitting upright. Now try the same exercise, but the other way round, with your left leg stretched out and your right one bent, reaching out towards your left foot.

This movement also originates in the Muladhara Chakra. When you have mastered it fully, you will find that you

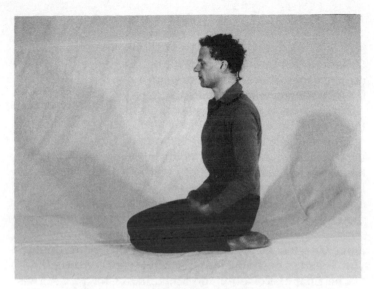

Photo 1

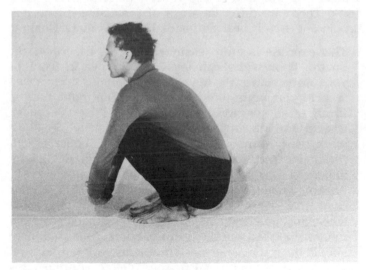

Photo 2

are able to touch the soles of your feet with your fingers. Relax into this position, and massage the places on your sole where the fingers naturally reach. Work for a while on any places that are sore or uncomfortable.

Now lie on your back, relax, and listen to your body. Feel the flow of energy.

This rest period should be as long as the exercise, and in a way it is just as active. By allowing everything to happen that needs to happen, you will find that a lot is going on in your body. Do not hold on to any thoughts and feelings that arise — let them go again.

At the end of the rest period breathe with your natural rhythm for about half a minute, tensing your anus muscles as you breathe out and relaxing them as you breathe in. Pause briefly after each outbreath.

The final exercise for the Muladhara Chakra is a twist called the Ardha-Matsendrasana, a classical yoga asana. You will find a description of it in every yoga book. There are different ways of practising this asana; this is one which best activates the Muladhara Chakra.

This exercise is more easily done than described. Sit on the floor with both legs straight out in front of you. Move your right leg up towards your body, crossing it over your left leg so that your right foot is firmly on the ground beside your left knee (Photo 3). Check that you are sitting straight, and feel the floor under you. Both buttocks should be in contact with the floor. Breathe deeply into your Muladhara Chakra, and as you breathe out twist your body to the right. Keeping your left arm straight, hold the ankle of your right foot with your left hand, at the same time stretching your right hand behind your back to touch the left hip with the back of the hand. Your shoulders should be in the same straight line as your left leg, and you can turn your head to the right to continue this line (Photo 4). Got it?

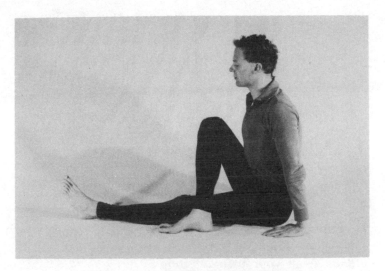

Photo 3: The Ardha-Matsendraasana (1)

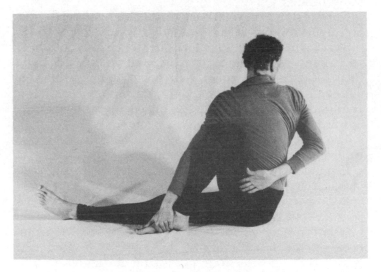

Photo 4: The Ardha-Matsendraasana (2)

You have now turned your spine from the os sacrum to the neck. While you are in this position, breathe deeply into your Muladhara Chakra. Relax in this position, and take note of what you can see behind you.

Now try doing this exercise the other way round, with your left foot beside your right knee. What can you see behind you now? Is it different from when you did it the first time? How does doing the exercise this way feel different from the first time?

When you are back in the starting position each time, let your fingers move over the soles of your feet, paying particular attention to the instep. You can press quite hard. It isn't important to know exactly where the reflexology points are — this knowledge can easily detract from your own intuition.

At the very end of the exercise, touch both your big toes. This is a Jin Shin Jyutzu technique, and helps to bring peace.

Now lie down on your back on the floor and relax, your arms lying relaxed beside your body. Watch your feelings.

Slowly turn on to your left side; touch the bottom of your spine with your right hand, and your Svadisthana Chakra, just about where your pubic hair is, with your left hand. Breathe deeply and feel the energy channels in your body. Imagine these pulsating energies being drawn upwards through the body.

The exercises for the Muladhara Chakra can be concluded with the following affirmation:

'I stand firmly within life, which I create lovingly and imaginatively.'

For anyone who is interested in the astrological connections, the Muladhara Chakra is symbolised by the Cancer-Capricorn axis. It is also possible to see a link between the four petals of the lotus associated with this chakra and the four phases of the moon.

If you would like to work creatively with this chakra,

you can do the following visualisation, and afterwards turn it into a painting. Visualise a square, immediately in front of us, which slowly turns into a cube. When you can see it clearly, visualise it turning slowly into a bright red, vibrating, flowing cubic form. Let this form dance. Return slowly from the visualisation, and paint what you have visualised.

THE SACRAL CHAKRA
SVADISTHANA

With the Svadisthana Chakra we connect with the astrological axis of Taurus-Scorpio, and the realm of sexuality. The six-petal lotus associated with this chakra relates to the 'Venus hexagram' — the upper and lower conjunction of Venus with the Sun in the zodiac.

You can begin your exercises with a meditation on the Tarot card number VI, The Lovers, sometimes called The Decision.

After meditating for at least fifteen minutes, you can start the first body exercise.

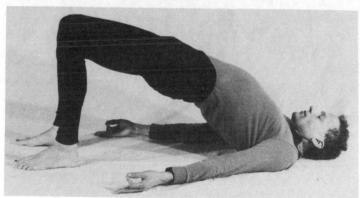

Photo 5

Lie down on your back and relax, and feel how your
body rests on the floor. Now bend your knees so that
your feet rest squarely on the ground. In time with
the rhythm of your breathing, lift your back from the
bottom upwards, vertebra by vertebra, until you are
only making contact with the floor with your feet,
shoulders and head (see Photo 5). Concentrate on the
Svadisthana Chakra and breathe into it, pausing
briefly after the outbreath. Do this exercise five
times, then relax, your knees still bent and your
feet touching each other, then let your knees fall to
each side.

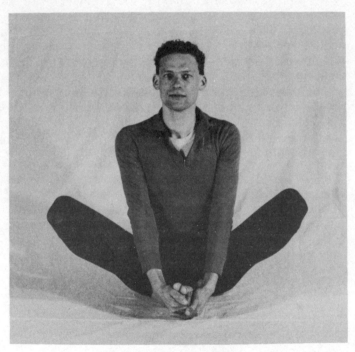

Photo 6: The Butterfly

The next exercise is called The Butterfly.

Sit on the floor with the soles of your feet touching each other. Bring your heels as near as possible to your body. Breathe in and stretch your back so that it is perfectly straight — this should raise your chest slightly. In time with your breathing, move your knees slowly up and down (Photo 6). Concentrate on the Svadisthana Chakra and try to maintain that concentration throughout the exercise. After a few minutes, end the exercise by bending your body down towards your feet, breathing out as you bend, then coming up again, breathing in as you do so. Now lie down on your back, breathe deeply and regularly, and feel the flow of energy in the lower part of your body.

During this exercise it is easy to massage the insteps of your feet with your thumbs — try it. In the arch on the inside of your feet you will find an important acupuncture point — SP4 (Spine 4), but see if you can find it before looking it up. After relaxing for a few minutes, move into the next exercise.

Sit on your heels, with your hands touching your knees. Breathe in deeply and, by lifting your chest a little and pushing it out, make your back concave (Photo 7). As you breathe out, push your back in the opposite direction, so it is now convex, letting your head fall gently forward (Photo 8). Concentrate on your Sacral Chakra and try to maintain this concentration throughout the exercise.

Do this exercise for one or two minutes, gradually speeding up the movement as you go from concave to convex and back again. After this exercise, lie down on your back and relax.

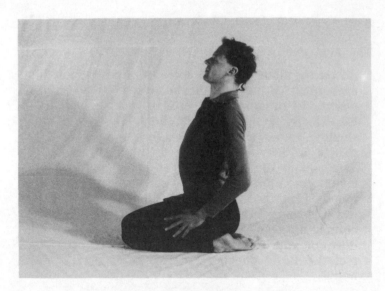

Photo 7

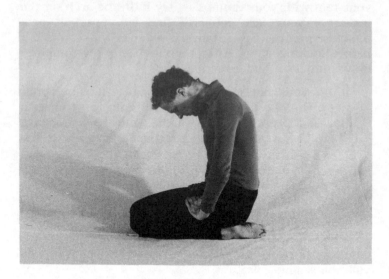

Photo 8

The next exercise is called The Cat.

Get down on the floor on your hands and knees, with your back parallel to the floor and your head lifted slightly. In this position breathe deeply in and out, pausing after each outbreath. Breathe into your Svadisthana Chakra. When you can feel the chakra very clearly (from its warmth, flow or whatever — these feelings are very subjective), concentrate on it. As you breathe in, arch your back as much as possible, and let your head drop loosely (Photo 9). As you breathe out, let your back fall towards the floor, moving your head up and back as far as it will go (Photo 10). By concentrating on the Sacral Chakra, you can move up and down in time with your breathing. Always pause after breathing out, and feel the flow of energy in the Svadisthana Chakra.

After this exercise, lie down flat on the floor on your back and relax, still concentrating on the Svadisthana Chakra, and watching your breathing without trying to control it. At first you should do this exercise for about three minutes, gradually extending it to about five. The longer you do it, the more clearly you will feel the energyin your Sacral Chakra, especially as you relax afterwards.

As you start to relax, ask yourself the following questions:

'Am I able to surrender?'

'Can I open myself to others?'

With these questions in your mind, let yourself fall deeper and deeper into this relaxed state, letting go of all resistance. If you feel fear, simply accept it.

After a while, you can decide to end this relaxation period. End it by stretching and yawning, since yawning always produces relaxation. If you want to, take this opportunity to write down what you have experienced.

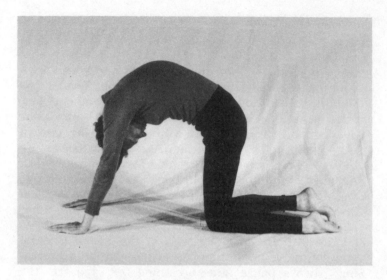

Photo 9

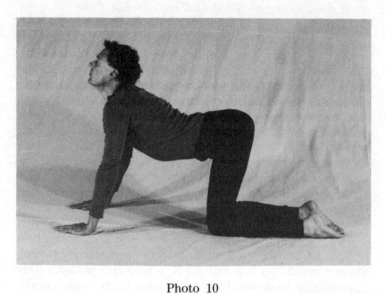

Photo 10

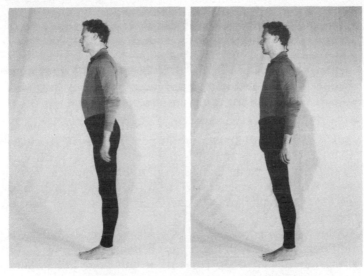

Photo 11   Photo 12

Now stand on the floor with your feet a little wider apart than the width of your shoulders. Let your arms drop by your sides and find a point straight ahead of you to focus on. As you breathe into your Svadisthana Chakra, push your pelvis hard backwards (Photo 11) concentrating all the time on your Sacral Chakra. As you breathe out again, push your pelvis hard forwards (Photo 12). After you have pushed forwards with the oubreath, always pause briefly before pushing backwards again. It is important for this exercise to have your feet firmly on the ground.

After working with this exercise for about three minutes, it should immediately be followed by the equivalent female movement.

Put your feet about the width of your shoulders apart and bend your knees slightly. Now rotate your pelvis

so that it makes a circle parallel to the floor. Start
very slowly and gradually make the movment more
energetic. Start by moving first to the right, then
change direction, all the time breathing in time with
your body movement. Find your own rhythm, and
keep concentrating on your Sacral Chakra.

It may help you if you visualise a warm orange point at
your Svadisthana Chakra while you do these exercises,
but that may take some practice, and to begin with you
should try the visualisation separately from the exercises. When you are able to do it, however, it will help
you to maintain your concentration on the Sacral
Chakra.

After these exercises, lie down on your back flat on
the floor and relax, being aware of your breathing. After
a few minutes of deep relaxation, put your left fingers
on the Svadisthana Chakra and the right fingers on the
Sahasrara Chakra. Maintain this position for a few
minutes, breathing deeply.

Now you might like to massage your hands. In classical yoga, sutras associate the Sacral Chakra with the
hands, particularly the palms of the hands. Look out for
points that are painful; massage these areas until the
pain changes.

In Red Tantra the Sacral Chakra is often stimulated
by the following exercise:

On an empty stomach, drink a glass of water, then
wait for an hour before passing water. When you
empty your bladder, control the stream of urine all
the time by alternately holding it and then letting it
go. When you are able to maintain this sort of control
over the muscles of the urethra (for women a little
below the clitoris, for men at the base of the penis),
you will be able to do this exercise without needing

to urinate. Holding your breath with half-filled lungs, you should be able alternately to tense and relax this muscle several times. This exercise also stimulates the Muladhara Chakra.

The affirmation for this chakra is:
'Opening myself to my surroundings gives me new possibilities for change.'

If you would like to work creatively with this chakra, visualise a large pyramid in which you can sit comfortably. Breathe deeply into your stomach, and as you breathe out, fill this pyramid with an orange mist that flows and circulates within the pyramid. You might like to paint this image.

THE NAVEL CHAKRA
MANIPURA

> *"What the centre holds is clear:*
> *What was at the beginning*
> *and what will be at the end."*
> Goethe *The Seat of East and West*

Everybody knows the story of St George and the dragon, and the picture of the patron saint of England slaying that ferocious beast is the subject of many paintings and stained glass windows. But there are also pictures in which a beautiful princess holds the dragon on a lead.

The dragon represents the wild animal, the drives and desires, in each of us. Typically the man, St George, strives to kill these drives and desires, but the woman does not attempt to kill the dragon, only to tame it. There is a famous Renaissannce painting of St George

Figure 8
St George and The Dragon

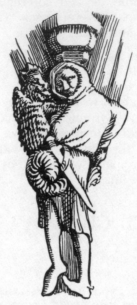

(from a drawing of a capital in Cley Church, Norfolk,
by Susan Lescelles)

the dragon by Paolo Uccello (1397-1475) in the National
Gallery — I can recommend taking this painting with its
archetypal symbolism as the subject of a meditation.

Start your work on the Manipura Chakra by meditating on the archetype of The Hermit, using Tarot card
number IX.

When we work with the Manipura Chakra, tremen-
dous energies are set free. Suppressed anger and
aggression often erupt, especially in group work, and
this is to be welcomed within reason.

In order to be prepared for this work, start with a
Tibetan cleansing ritual, which should be performed

using the mantra 'Yaman Taka Ant Fat'. The mantra
helps to keep the movements in rhythm; the meaning of
the words is less important than their sound, though
because Westerners always like to know the literal
meaning of things, a rough translation is: 'The Way;
Death; The End; The Inexpressible.'

In Tibetan, 'Yamantaka' is the feared one who
overcame death. According to Govinda[3], he is none
other than the compassionate Avalokitesvara "who in
his role as the judge of death allows those who have
gone astray to look into the mirror of truth."

Intoning the mantra 'Yaman Taka Ant Fat', touch
both sides of your body with your hands, starting at
your ankles and moving upwards to the shoulders.
Then, when you reach the word 'Fat', you throw your
arms up and out. Let the rhythm become faster and
faster, imagining that with the final 'Fat' you are
throwing away everything that you do not like about
yourself. According to eye-witnesses, Tibetan monks
do this cleansing ritual in a very abandoned way —
you could try doing it like this too. When you are
totally exhausted by this movement, hold your arms
up and imagine a bright ball above you, into which you
have now put everything you don't like about
yourself. Look at this ball very carefully, and slowly
start to play with it. Your arms should still be
stretched upwards, and you get the energy to hold
them up from the Manipura Chakra. Breathe deeply
into this chakra without pausing. When you have
played with this ball of light for a while, welcome it
back into your body, together with all the things
about yourself that you find difficult, and let your
arms fall to your sides in a relaxed way. Remain
standing, and with your eyes closed, take some time
to tune into your body.

During this cleansing, the movement of the hands up the body has a special purpose. It has the effect of de-energising the body, protecting it against dangerously high levels of vibration, and calming it deeply.[4] Tender caressing helps quietly to desensitise the body. The next exercise is a classical yoga asana, the Paschimottanasana, or The Pincers.

Lie down on the floor, fully stretched out and relaxed, with your eyes closed and your arms beside your body. With full concentration, breathe deeply and slowly into your Manipura Chakra. Slowly circle your hands and arms outwards on the floor until they meet above your head. Now stretch and make yourself as long as possible, and then relax (Photo 13).

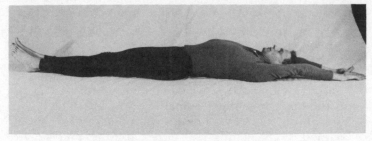

Photo 13: Paschimottanasana (1)

All your breathing and concentration should be fixed on your Manipura Chakra. Now lift your arms slowly, keeping them together, until they are vertically above your head — your head should remain motionless on the floor. Open your eyes, and bring your arms slowly down until your hands are lying on your thighs, lifting your head at the same time, but keeping your shoulders on the ground — this is important. Now, moving your hands slowly down towards your feet, lift your back from the floor vertebra by vertebra. Ideally you should eventually be able to put your forehead on your knees and your chest on your thighs, and hold the soles of your feet with your hands, finding a pressure point there and pressing it. When your body is pressed together in this way like a pair of pincers, relax and breathe deeply and slowly into your Manipura Chakra, without pausing in your breathing (Photo 14).

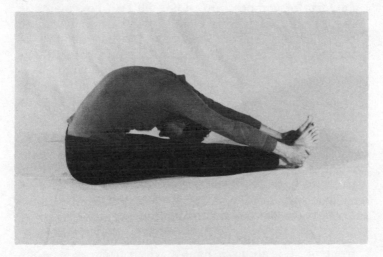

Photo 14: Paschimottanasana (2)

When you do this exercise, do not strain yourself. Only reach as far and for as long as you can comfortably hold the tension in your body. Do not seesaw in the effort to reach your toes. It is not important to see how far you can reach!

What feelings come up for you as you bend your body?
Are you aware of any of the symbolism of bending like
this?

Paschimotta means 'rising in the East'. Laya Yoga
practitioners use this position to allow the life energies
(Kundalini) rise up the spine (the back represents the
West, or Paschima) into the back of your head, but even
the 'average' student of yoga can feel the flow of
energy up the back if this position is held for long
enough.

Stay in this position for about a minute, then return
to your former position, doing all the movements in
the reverse order. Now relax, lying on your back and
being aware of your feelings. Do not identify or
interfere with your feelings — simply watch them.
After a couple of minutes, send any sound which feels
appropriate into the Manipura Chakra, and feel the
vibrations in your body. Play with this sound. You
might try the mantra 'Yang', but it is more important to find a sound which exactly expresses your
present mood.

The Manipura Chakra is associated with fire, and
astrologically with the Sun. Fire and the Sun represent
the light which allows us to see things. The next
exercise is a glass bead meditation.[5]

Take two glass marbles and put them on the floor in
front of you, about a hand's width from each other.
Sit in a meditative position about six feet away from
them, and concentrate on the marbles. Squint or
cross your eyes very slightly, and try to see clearly a
third marble in the middle between the two real
marbles. When you can see the third marble clearly,
breathe deeply without pausing into your Manipura
Chakra, and hold that image. Concentrate fully on
your Manipura Chakra, since each lapse in concentra-

tion tends to cause the third marble to divide in two.
If this happens, just gently bring them back together
again. Relax into the centre of your body.

At the end of this exercise, sit on your heels with a
straight spine and concentrate your breathing into your
Manipura Chakra, ready for the next exercise.

Still sitting in this position, move your pelvis forwards as you breathe out, backwards as you breathe
in. Maintain the rhythm of your breathing. Try to feel
the centre of gravity of your body. Do this for about
three minutes, then lie down on your back and relax.
Put your right hand on your Manipura Chakra and
your left hand on your Sahasrara Chakra. After a while
you may feel a pulsing between the two points.
Concentrate on this feeling.

While I have been living in old houses with big fire-
places, I have enjoyed meditating on fire. This is very
easy. It simply involves sitting for half an hour in frontof
the flames, letting your feelings rise with them. When
you have practised this for a while, you can meditate in
this way for up to a couple of hours.

To begin with your eyes may hurt and water. Don't
worry if you start to cry — this is a stage that must be
gone through when old feelings of hurt and pain come up
after doing the previous exercises. You will suddenly
find that your spirit starts to move more easily, that
you can readily identify with the changing patterns of
the flames.

This is a powerful cleansing exercise, as well as being
an excellent exercise for training your concentration. It
is said that Nostradamus received his visions of the
future while using this technique, which he learned from
people who were in touch with the Cathars.

It may sound simple, but it takes a great deal of
practice to master this meditation, and you can gain a

great deal from it.

To finish your work with the Manipura Chakra, use the affirmation for this chakra, which is:

'I am open, and fight in a positive way.'

Astrologically speaking, this chakra stimulates the Aries-Libra axis. The ten petals of the lotus associated with this chakra relate to the double pentagram of Venus.

If you continue to feel inhibitions and resistances while doing the exercises with this chakra, see if there is any residual aggression which is creating these blocks. You may not feel this in your Manipura Chakra itself — aggression often lodges in the shoulders, for example. If you do find such tensions, follow what your body is telling you and move your body accordingly. Always think of the exercises I have given simply as suggestions, which you can modify as you need to.

For a creative visualisation on this chakra, imagine a circle around your navel which slowly changes into a cylinder. With your breath, slowly fill this cylinder with a shiny pale yellow substance which streams in and out of it. Play with the energy in the cylinder. Paint a picture of it if you would like to.

The classical visualisation of the Manipura Chakra is a golden ball. This visualisation is traditionally used as a protection meditation.

THE HEART CHAKRA
ANAHATA

In astrological terms, we have here the Leo-Aquarius axis. The twelve petals of the lotus associated with this chakra represent the twelve conjunctions and oppositions of the Sun and Moon.

The Heart Chakra can be entered with a meditation on Tarot card number XII, The Hanged Man. At the level of the Heart Chakra, all meditation which looks at your dark side with the light of love must be seen as positive.

The courage provided by this perspective allows you to distance yourself a little from your dark side, so that you may acknowledge it without having to act it out. If you always act out your dark side you are simply giving it more power, and you will stay on the level of darkness. Aggression is a good example. Acting out your aggression will always attract the dark in the form of counter-aggression. If you can simply be aware of the aggression within you, this is the first step towards acceptance and dealing with the feelings (see Figure 8 again). You cannot follow the freeing of the Manipura Chakra with the freeing of the Anahata Chakra until you have dealt with your dark side. Unacknowledged hatred always has the power to block the Anahata Chakra.

At the level of the Manipura Chakra, the question was how to deal with aggression. Here at the level of the Heart Chakra the question is: How can I deal with my love? This question should be uppermost in your mind during all the exercises related to this chakra.

A very powerful meditation for the Heart Chakra is practised in the Eastern Orthodox Church. It dates back to fourteenth century ritual from the monastic tradition of Mount Athos in Greece, and in particular from the teachings of St Seraphim, who said "The Kingdom of God is within the human heart."

Sit down in any meditation position, and visualise your heart until you can see it clearly. When you have a clear picture, repeat one of the following prayers as a sort of mantra: either 'Christ have mercy upon me, a poor sinner', or 'Lord have pity upon me'. This prayer should be thought of as vibrating deeply into your heart.

Tradition says that this mantric prayer contains a power far greater than its words alone would suggest. If we think of sin as an attitude of limiting egotism, of being unnecessarily attached, this exercise can open us up again. Concentrating on the heart during chakra work always has the effect of opening you up. By concentrating on your heart and its movements you can see all your rigidity (the 'evil') being released, and your true self becoming open and harmonious once more.

Before going on with more individual exercises, I would like to describe an exercise that is done with a partner — this seems entirely appropriate, since the Anahata Chakra is after all about overcoming distances.

Both partners should lie down beside each other on their backs and relax, breathing deeply according to their own natural rhythm. Both should try to be aware of their heartbeat. After breathing like this for a while, each of you should reach out and place a hand gently on the other's Heart Chakra. Keep breathing calmly and regularly, gradually bringing your breathing into synchronisation with each other. Do not force this — just let it happen. Can you allow it? Is there any resistance? Can you say when you want to stop?

This exercise should be done for about fifteen minutes. Take a little time to talk about it afterwards. Now to the individual exercises.[6]

Stand up straight with your feet about the width of your shoulders apart, and breathe deeply, without pausing, into your Heart Chakra. Feel comfortable about where and how you are standing. Now raise your arms above your head and bend back as far as you can, until you can see the world upside down. Breathe

into your Heart Chakra and be aware of your heartbeat (Photo 15).

Some people see sparks dancing in front of their eyes
when they do this exercise. Don't worry — it is simply
the unaccustomed strain of the body. When you have
practised this exercise for a while, you might be able to
transform these sparks into a greenish veil, but this
needs some experience. At the end of this exercise, relax
by letting your body fall forwards with your arms
dangling loose. Now you are ready for the second part of
this exercise.

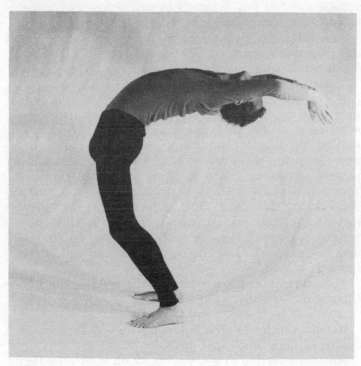

Photo 15

Bring yourself very slowly — vertebra by vertebra — back to the upright position. Now interlock the fingers of your hands together behind your back, then lean backwards again as far as possible, at the same time pushing your arms, interlocked fingers upwards, away from your back. Breathe deeply and regularly. Hold this position for as long as is comfortable, then as with the last exercise, let your body fall forwards to relax.

Be careful with this exercise if you have any circulation difficulties. When you first do these exercises, don't be surprised if you find yourself breathless — this is quite normal. The breathlessness will go as you practise.

Now relax deeply, concentrate on your heartbeat, and say: 'My heart beats quietly and regularly.' Place your left hand on your heart chakra, your right hand on your Sahasrara Chakra, and let all your feelings come up.

If you are unable to feel your heart during these exercises, my experience suggests that it may well have something to do with unresolved issues about your mother. If this is the case, humanistic psychology provides many ways of working with your 'internalised mother syndrome'. If you want to work on it by yourself, working with your dreams is a good way of approaching the issue. How dependent is your dream ego on the love and attention of your mother, or of women in general? How dependent are you on attention and recognition? How does your dream ego behave towards women?

The affirmation for working at the level of the Heart Chakra is:

'Thy will be done.'

It is worth meditating on the old-established trinity of faith, hope and love.

An easy exercise to get you in touch with your Heart Chakra, and one that you can do whenever and wherever you want, is to pause for a moment, doing nothing, and checking that you can feel your heartbeat. A useful symbol for the Heart Chakra is a red rose, which you can imagine putting over the chakra. See if you can feel any subtle change as you do this.

The visualisation exercise that goes with the Heart Chakra, which you may like to express artistically, is to imagine a green cross in front of your eyes, with equal-length arms. When you can see this cross clearly, let it grow until it is as big as you are. Now cover it with streamers of green energy which come from your breathing, and whirl around the cross. You can paint this if you would like to.

THE THROAT CHAKRA
VISHUDDHA

> *"Screaming did not make me mad,*
> *Nor doubt nor being questioned.*
> *How could humans devils know*
> *Had the devil ne'er existed?"*
> Goethe

Work on the Throat Chakra begins with a meditation on the archetype of The Devil: Tarot card number XV. You might find it useful to read the chapter about the archetype of the dark angel in Sallie Nicholls' book *Jung and the Tarot: An Archetypal Journey*.[7]

Many of the well-known classical yoga asanas affect the Throat Chakra, and this makes a great deal of sense in a culture which is overly determined by language, using the throat as the centre of communication.

The Vishuddha Chakra is also called Bharati-Sthana — 'the dwelling-place of the goddess of language'.

If you are alone and can spare the time, it can be very useful to try to write your autobiography in the form of a fairy tale. Even more effective is to tell it in this

form to a friend. What is important is to tell it
spontaneously, without thinking it out too carefully.

Which character from fairy tale matches best with
the way you see yourself and your life? Is there a happy
ending? What is the moral of the story?

But now to the physical exercises. I want to suggest
three classical yoga exercises, which can be combined
well as a series: Halasana (The Plough), Sarwangasana
(The Shoulder Stand), and Matsyaasana (The Fish).
Before you start these exercises, take a few minutes to
exercise your neck by moving your head sideways, then
back and forth.

Sit down on the floor with your spine straight (it does
not have to be a lotus or half-lotus position — any
position where you can hold your back straight for a
few minutes is fine). Now slowly move your head from
side to side and backwards and forwards. Do not roll
your head — the neck joints are not constructed for a
rolling movement and you can hurt yourself. Stick to
sideways   and   back-and-forward   movements.
Change the direction often, and gradually get faster;
then slow down again, breathing deeply into any
places that feel tense. Now lie down on the floor and
relax. Keeping your head on the floor and your upper
spine as straight as possible, move your chin slightly
towards your neck. Concentrate on your Throat
Chakra and breathe deeply into it, pausing slightly
after each inbreath (it can be very relaxing to imagine
this chakra as blue). Now slowly lift your legs, keeping
them straight, until they touch the floor behind your
head (Photo 16) — this is The Plough. In this
position, your chin is pressing the point where your
thyroid gland is situated. Breathe deeply into this
point, pausing after each inbreath, and feel the energies in your thyroid gland. Now return slowly to your
starting position, rolling back vertebra by vertebra.

Now relax, lying on your back with your eyes closed. Concentrate on your throat chakra and feel how the breath streams in and out through your throat.

The Halasana is very important for those who sit for most of the day. This exercise improves body symmetry, and enhances the harmony of the whole body. The back muscles will be strengthened by the stretching, becoming strong and moving easily. At the same time it will balance the positive and negative energy streams in your body.

If you do not live in a house with thin walls, use this opportunity to shout as loud as you can at the end of

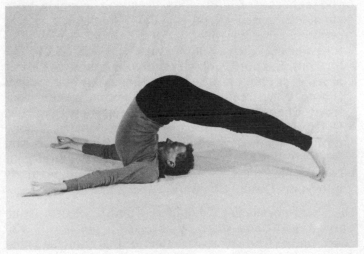

Photo 16: Halasana, The Plough

the relaxation period, imagining your throat becoming wider and more relaxed.

If the shouting makes you hoarse, this is a sign that the energy is not flowing freely through your Throat Chakra. You can loosen the chakra by sending a

humming sound into your throat, imagining it widening
and opening up your throat.
Ask yourself how you use language. Do you commun-
icate openly and honestly?
The second of the classical exercises for this chakra is
The Shoulder Stand.

Lie down on your back and relax. Slowly lift your legs,
keeping them straight, but keep your back on the
ground. It is important that you do not start to lift
your back yet, since you could damage your fifth
lumbar vertebra and the connected discs. When your
legs are nearly vertical, stretched towards the ceiling,
you can start to lift your back too, keeping your
shoulders and neck on the floor. Remaining in this
position, relax your feet and legs (do not stretch your
toes towards the ceiling because this will add to the
tension). Support yourself with your hands and lower
arms, your chin pressed hard against your upper chest
(Photo 17). Breathe deeply and regularly into your
Heart Chakra, moving your diaphragm energetically.
Don't worry if your throat feels tense — this is quite
normal. Come down again in the same way as you
went up, but in reverse. When you are lying on your
back again, relax by breathing deeply and regularly
into your Throat Chakra.

The Sarwangasana (Shoulder Stand) comes from
'Sarva-Anga-Uttana-Asana', or 'the position with
raised limbs'. The particular effect of this exercise isthat
the cosmic vibrations affect the body the opposite
way round to normal, which has a harmonising effect.
Women who are menstruating should not attempt this
exercise.
    It is always recommended that you do The Fish after
either or both of the previous two exercises, since it is
an exercise which bends the spine in the opposite
direction, freeing and stretching the neck.

Sit with your spine straight in a meditation position. Bend your head slowly backwards, supporting yourself with your elbows on the ground. Let you head fall backwards, and try to touch the ground with your head as near as possible to the Sahasrara Chakra, thus stretching your throat and neck. Breathe deeply into your Vishuddha Chakra. Now take the supporting elbows away and rest only on your head and lower body (Photo 18). It is important at this stage to breathe very deeply. If you have a strong spine you can place both your arms — stretched out — behind your

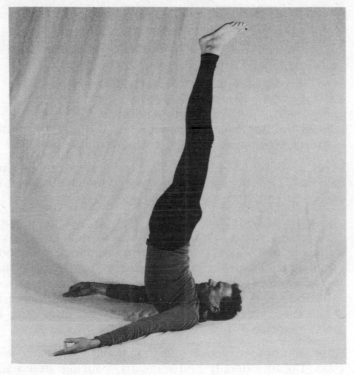

Photo 17: Sarwangasana; The Shoulder Stand

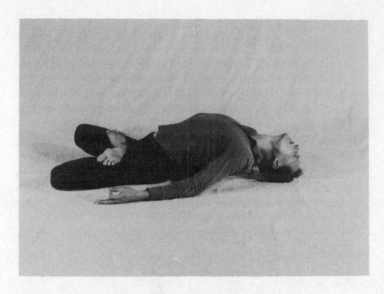

Photo 18: Matsyasana; The Fish

head on the floor. This improves the effects of the exercise because it helps to expand the chest.

If you are interested in working more intensively on this chakra I would recommend the following shouting exercises which come from bioenergetics:

Stand up straight, with your feet the width of your shoulders apart. Pressing both your fists into your back at about the level of your waist, bend your body slowly backwards. Bend your knees slightly. Hold this position for as long as possible. After a while you will begin to feel a trembling. Let this trembling increase, and then shout to help reduce the tension. Stay in this position for several minutes.

After all these exercises, lie down on your back and relax. Breathe deeply and regularly, pausing after each inbreath. Now place your left hand slowly on your Vishuddha Chakra and your right hand on your Sahasrara Chakra. Let the feelings come up — you might like to write them down afterwards.

The affirmations for this chakra are:
   'I approach other people openly.'
   'My language is clear.'
   'My communication is honest and direct.'

As a visualisation exercise for this chakra, close your eyes and imagine a goblet or grail. Fill this grail by breathing into it a blue liquid that swirls around inside it. When you can see this image clearly, pour out the blue liquid, which becomes a blue mist in the surrounding atmosphere. Taste the liquid. See yourself becoming blue. You can paint this imagine if you want.

Astrologically speaking, we are dealing at this level with the Gemini-Sagittarius axis. With the sixteen petals of the lotus of this chakra you might like to meditate on the eight loops of Mars during its two phases.

THE THIRD EYE
AJNA

Work on the Ajna Chakra starts with a meditation on Tarot card number XVIII, The Moon.

Light a candle, set it in front of you at eye level, and stare at it. Before your eyes start to water, close them and concentrate on the after-image of the candle. After a few minutes open your eyes very slightly. Does the golden light you can now see come from the candle or from you? Where does it come from?

Sit in a meditation position with your spine straight and sing an 'Aum' which vibrates in your Third Eye.

Try bombarding your Third Eye from inside your head
with a variety of different sounds.

Now sit quietly and concentrate on your Ajna Chakra.
For a few minutes try to feel the point between your
eyebrows where the Third Eye is located as clearly as
you can. You are now ready for the first body exercise.

Support yourself with your arms and let your head fall
backwards so that your Ajna Chakra points upwards
towards the ceiling or the sky. Breathe deeply and
regularly into the chakra, pausing briefly after each
inbreath. Do this for a few minutes, then move your
head slowly back to the upright position. Feel the
energy in your Third Eye. Then let your head fall
backwards again as before and breathe in. Hold that
breath in your chest, making your chest as broad as
possible, letting the Prana energy rise up to your
Third Eye. Now breathe out again. Do this nine times.
Finally, lie down on your back and relax, for about the
same length of time as it took you to do the exercise.
Let yourself fall into complete relaxation.

The next exercise is based on one called 'Left Brain
versus Right Brain', which was originally developed by
Robert Masters and Jean Houston.[8]

Sit comfortably, supporting yourself against something if you prefer. Sit really comfortably, and feel
happy. Close your eyes and relax. Think of what you
would tell your brain if you could communicate
directly with it right now. What would you say? Wake
up your brain. Produce a sound, and send it into the
right hemisphere of your brain. Let it vibrate there.
Fill the whole of your right hemisphere with that
sound. Feel it tickling inside your right brain. Now do
the same with your left hemisphere. I find that this
part of the exercise works best with a humming
sound. Then relax. After a few minutes visualise the

number '1' in your left hemisphere and the letter 'A' in your right hemisphere. When you can see this clearly, move on to visualise '2' in the left hemisphere and 'B' in the right. Continue with this exercise until you reach number '26' and letter 'Z'. Now relax for about three minutes. Breathe deeply into your Ajna Chakra, pausing after each inbreath. Now go on with this exercise, doing the same as before but ths time visualising the letters in the left hemisphere and the numbers in the right. Now relax again, breathing into your Ajna Chakra with a pause after the inbreath. After a few minutes, imagine the sun rising in your right hemisphere and setting in the left. After this, imagine the moon rising in the left hemisphere and setting in the right. Now see what images arise for you in relation to each of the hemispheres — try playing with these pictures. Imagine looking at your left hemisphere with your right eye, and at your right hemisphere with your left eye. Now let everything go and relax. Open your eyes, get up, and walk slowly round your room or garden. Enjoy being fully awake; enjoy the vividness of your impressions.

If you feel tense after this exercise, you have probably pushed yourself too hard. Try to be more relaxed next time you do the exercise, or only do part of the exercise. The whole point is to enjoy it and feel more awake at the end! To do this exercise properly you need to take at least forty-five minutes. It is important to take it slowly.

Now lie down again and relax. Concentrate on your Ajna Chakra. After a few minutes put the index and middle fingers of your left hand on your Ajna Chakra, and the same fingers of your right hand on your Sahasrara Chakra. Let the feelings come up that want to.

Now get up and sit in front of a mirror. Look at your
Third Eye for about ten minutes, then lie down again
and relax. End these exercises with an 'Aum', letting it
vibrate in your Third Eye. Afterwards you might like to
meditate for a while on the theme of duality — duality
in yourself, duality in the world.

The affirmations for this level are:

'As above, so below.'

'I follow my inner guidance.'

In connection with all exercises to do with the Third
Eye, the Sufis recommend putting a little sandalwood
oil on the chakra.

A visualise exercise to go with this chakra is to
visualise a violet triangle pointing upwards, a little
above your eye level. When you can see this image
clearly, put another similar triangle above it with its
point downwards. Now combine both triangles to form
a six-pointed star (Solomon's Seal). Let this star
rotate, and see violet clouds streaming from the points
of the star. Play with these clouds. Paint them if you
would like to.

Astrologically speaking, this level relates to the
Virgo-Pisces axis.

THE CROWN CHAKRA
SAHASRARA

The level of the thousandfold lotus can no longer be
reached within the teacher-pupil relationship. The
exercises I give here can only provide the basis for
developing your own individual exercises, giving you a
direction and a few ideas. It is doubtful whether you can
in fact reach this level using exercises at all. The best
exercise — and one which is true for all the chakras — is

to live your daily life as awarely as possible.

Meditating on Tarot card number XXI — The Universe — can help to lead you into this realm beyond language. Lie down on your back, relax, and breathe into your Sahasrara Chakra. Listen to your body and your intuition, which will tell you how best to relax. Follow this intuition even if seems strange and inappropriate.

Breathe according to your natural rhythm, and imagine that you are breathing in through your Third Eye and out through your Sahasrara Chakra. Imagine too that with each outbreath through your Crown Chakra you are straightening your spine. As you breathe out, you may like to visualise a purple stream of energy flowing out of your Crown Chakra.

There are no affirmations to accompany this chakra, since it is beyond language. Here, however, are some visualisations which have helped me to gain a glimpse of what the Sahasrara Chakra is all about.

Close your eyes and breathe deeply and regularly, lifting the air up from your Muladhara Chakra and breathing it out through your Sahasrara Chakra. Transform this stream of air into a stream of water, which becomes stiller and stiller. Now imagine that on this water is floating a lotus with eight pinkish or pure white petals. Sit yourself in the middle of this flower. Paint this picture, and use it as a mandala to meditate on for three days. Then burn it and let the wind carry the ashes away.

Sit in a meditation position with your spine straight. Imagine that every time you breathe in you are taking in energy, and every time you breathe out the energy rises up your back, falls down through your front, and rises back up your spine again, leaving your body through the Sahasrara Chakra. Now visualise a lotus straight ahead of you, which grows more and more petals. Let these petals slowly change into all the colours of the rainbow. Paint this picture and meditate on it for three days, afterwards burning it and scattering the ashes to the wind.

Another visualisation exercise for this chakra is to imagine an enormous flame, with yourself in the middle of it. And that is about all that can be said about the Sahasrara Chakra!

Om Mani Padme Hum

1. I use the Mertz-Struck Tarot for these exercises, published in Interlaken in 1981.

2. For this exercise see Chapter 3.

3. Govina, Lama Anagarika *The Way of the White Clouds* Rider, 1984.

4. This can be seen in such customs as beating people with birch branches in the sauna.

5. Pennington, George *Little Manual for Players of the Glass Bead Game* Element, 1984.

6. For other exercises see an article by Yogi Bhajan in *Hologramm* magazine, November 1984.

7. Nichols, Sallie *Jung and Tarot: The Archetypal Journey* Weiser, U.S.A., 1981.

8. Houston, Jean *The Possible Human* Tarcher, U.S.A., 1982; Masters, Robert *Consciousness Expansion for Body and Spirit*.

10
Exercises for
All or Several
of the Chakras

Once you have tried out all the exercises for the individual chakras at least once, you will probably begin to experiences slight changes and shifts in your everyday life. Now is the time to introduce some further exercises which can stimulate more than one chakra at a time. When I work with a particular chakra I always start by doing one of these exercises first.

The decision about which chakra to work with on a particular day usually depends on the experiences I have had in relating to other people. Just at the moment, for example, I am having problems opening myself up to other people. The people I live with have pointed this out to me; I am afraid that I might lose my freedom, so I have tended to deal with it by keeping my distance and being rather cold. I fight against being tied down, and when this happens I always feel tense in my left shoulder. My reason tells me that fighting the potential for deeper relationships may lose me freedom rather than gaining it.

When this happens it is clear that I need to work with

my Anahata Chakra. Before I do this, however, I lie down
on the floor and breathe deeply and regularly into each
chakra in turn, starting with the Muladhara Chakra. I
breathe into each chakra for as long as it takes to feel it
clearly, then I go on to the next. When people start
with chakra work, many find that it helps to send a
sound into each chakra.

Now I would like to describe three further exercises
which are helpful after you have been working with your
chakras for a while.

The 'I Am' Exercise

Sit in a meditative position with your spine straight.
Breathe in deeply, imagining that you are breathing in
through the Ajna Chakra. As you breathe out, say 'I' in
a loud voice, visualising that sound together with the
breath that makes it come out of your Sahasrara
Chakra. This stretches and straightens your spine.

When you have completely emptied your lungs,
breathe in again through your Ajna Chakra, and as you
breathe out again through your Sahasrara Chakra, say
'Am' loudly, letting the 'm' vibrate right down your
spine. When it reaches the bottom of your spine, hold
the energy by tensing your anus muscles a little.

Do this exercise three times.

It is important when you do the 'I Am' exercise to
hold the energy in the body so it can work from the
inside. When the 'm' sound falls, do not let the energy
leave the body through your anus, but hold it inside you.

It is only the vibrations you hold inside the body that
can help to form you from inside.

The Yoni Mudra

This is a classical exercise of Laya Yoga, with some of my
own modifications. It is explained in the yoga scriptures,

the Gerandas, as follows: 'In the yoga sitting position
the sage closes his ears, eyes, nose and mouth with the
thumb, index finger, middle finger, ring finger and little
finger. He breathes in Prana with the Kaki-Mudra,
fuses it with the energy of the Apana, and using the
mantra "Hum Hamsa", concentrates on the six psychic
centres in their correct order.'

In this way the Kundalini rises to the Sahasrara
Chakra where sun- and moon-breathing, Shiva and
Shakti are one. If you can work on this exercise in its
classical form for a year — with a good teacher — it is
said that you can attain eternal life and overcome the
death of your body.

Well, I am not too much concerned in overcoming the
death of the body, so I will describe a similar but less
demanding exercise which will help you to concentrate
on your chakras.

You will find other forms of the Yoni Mudra described
in Roman Blair's book on Laya Yoga.[1]

Sit in the meditation position with your spine
straight, relax, and breathe deeply. Now close your ears
with your thumbs, your eyes with your index fingers,
and place your middle fingers at the sides of your nose,
so you can open and close your right and left nostrils
alternately. With the other two fingers of each hand,
hold your lips together.

Now breathe deeply into the right nostril, closing the
left one with your middle finger. Breathe deeply until
you can feel it in your Muladhara Chakra. Breathe out
through the right nostril, then close it with your middle
finger. Now breathe deeply into the Muladhara Chakra
through your left nostril, until it feels really warm.

Now do the same with each chakra until you reach
the Sahasrara Chakra, then do it in reverse until you
reach the Muladhara Chakra once more.

When you have mastered this exercise, you could try

visualising the following colours at each of the chakras:
Muladhara — red
Svadisthana — orange
Manipura — yellow
Anahata — green
Vishuddha — blue
Ajna — violet
Sahasrara — purple
By visualising these qualities of colour[2] you will tune
into the different qualities of feeling that are assoc-
iated with these colours.

Doing this exercise will help you to harmonise your
energies in your seven energy centres, which will help
you live your daily life in a more harmonious way.

If you do this exercise on its own, rather than
integrated with other exercises, lie down afterwards,
relax and concentrate on the flow of energy in your
body.

The Small Middle Line

This is an exercise developed from Jin Shin Jyutzu. I
have used this exercise many times both for myself and
in groups, and it nearly always works. It seems to be
independent of the level of concentration it is given,
and of the surroundings.

You can either do it yourself, or have another person
do it on you, which can sometimes be even more
effective.

Step 1
Place the fingers of your right hand on your Sahasrara
Chakra, and the fingers of your left hand on your Ajna
Chakra. Keep your fingers there until you can feel a pulse
quite clearly in both places. This combination of points
seems to induce calm and concentration, and help the
intuition. The theory of Jin Shin Jyutzu says that it also
helps against senility!

Step 2
Keep the fingers of your right hand on the Sahasrara Chakra, but place the fingers of your left hand on the tip of your nose. Keep them there until you can feel a clear pulse. This combination of points seems to harmonise the Ida, Pingala and Sushumna energy flows, keeping your actions, feelings and meditation in harmony. In Jin Shin Jyutzu theory, this combination of points harmonises the surface energy streams of your body. Some chakra theories say that the Ida and Pingala 'nerves' end at the tip of the nose, while the Sushumna 'nerve' ends at the Sahasrara Chakra.

Step 3
Keep the fingers of your right hand on the Sahasrara Chakra, but move those of your left hand to the Vishuddha Chakra. Again, keep them there until you can feel a clear pulse. This relaxes the Vishuddha Chakra and harmonises your thinking and feeling. Jin Shin Jyutzu theory says that these points balance out the rising and falling energy streams in your body.

Step 4
Keeping the fingers of your right hand on the Sahasrara Chakra, move those of the left to your Anahata Chakra. This dissolves restlessness and hatred. This combination can be used to treat 'sorrow of the Heart Chakra'[3], which is the basis of the many psychosomatic illnesses that originate in internalised sorrow. Jin Shin Jyutzu theory says that this combination of points harmonises the hormones and frees the emotions.

Step 5
The fingers of the right hand are now placed on your back at the base of the spine (this is easiest if you lie on your left side); the fingers of your left hand on the Svadisthana Chakra. The combination reduces fear. Jin Shin Jyutzu theory says that it can reduce even the tightest tension.

All these combinations of touching can be done through your clothes, and all should be held until you can feel a definite pulse. When it takes a long time to feel the pulse, it can be a guide to the areas you need to work with.

Contrary to normal Jin Shin Jyutzu practice, I sometimes do these exercises in a sitting meditation pose, staring at a candle. This gives me a real feeling of strength, which I can maintain after the meditation as I go out into the world.

If you do Jin Shin Jyutzu lying down, rest afterwards for a few minutes and listen to your body.

Some people see dreamlike pictures during Jin Shin Jyutzu exercises, which can be worked with just like real dreams. These images can often provide a clue to which chakras need to be worked with.

1. Blair, Roman *Yoga for the Family* Sydney, 1966. See exercises 8 and 9.

2. The Tibetan system uses different colours, which you might prefer:

Muladhara — yellow
Svadisthana — white
Manipura — red
Anahata — green
Vishuddha — smokelike or translucent green

My system of colours follows Goethe's colour theory, and is based on the idea that the qualities of the colours reflect the qualities of the associated chakras.

3. According to chakra theory, there are two classes of psychosomatic illness: one is to do with the sorrow of the Heart Chakra, the other with blocks in the Manipura Chakra.

11
Conclusion

When you have been practising chakra exercises regularly for some time, and have a much better awareness of your behaviour (and particularly your subconscious habits), it is important to move to the next level with your exercises, or even to stop doing them altogether. If you listen to it carefully, your body will tell you when it is time to stop (usually somewhere between three and five years) — by this time you should find that the exercises and your daily life are virtually inseparable anyway.

You will have reached the next level when you recognise that your life has become the perfect exercise in itself. Then all these exercises will be seen for what they are — steps on the path to an understanding of yourself.

12
Bach Flower Remedies in Chakra Work

Alongside your chakra work you can also use the traditional high-potency homoeopathic remedies, or the Bach Flower Remedies.

If you can recall our model of vibrations, we saw that each chakra reflects the entire vibrational field with its own vibration. Both Bach Flower Remedies and homoeopathic remedies work by having a vibration which resonates with the vibration of the individual chakras, thus changing the overall vibration field. These remedies can thereby help to free the energies in a blocked chakra, transforming the kinetic energy back into potential energy. This results in an energy flow in the whole field, meaning that all the other chakras will be stimulated in turn.

I rarely work with homoeopathic remedies because I find them too complicated, and because I know very little about them. I do, however, use the Bach Flower Remedies a lot, and this chapter explains how you can use them to complement your chakra work.

J.T.C.—K

The Muladhara Chakra

Cherry plum	6	Learning to let go.
Clematis	9	Grounding.
Gorse	13	Integration of joy and sorrow.
Pine	24	Taking responsibility for your life.
Sweet chestnut	30	Trusting your own development

The Svadisthana Chakra

Crab apple	10	Getting rid of what you cannot digest.
Elm	11	Turning your ideas into reality.
Mimulus	20	Enjoying freedom within fixed structures.
Oak	22	Surrender.
Rock water	27	Discipline with release.
Vervain	31	Accepting others.
Wild rose	37	Taking part in life fully and joyfully.

The Manipura Chakra

Aspen	2	Overcoming fear.
Hornbeam	17	Being able to achieve personal goals.
Impatiens	18	Patience.
Larch	19	Self-awareness.
Scleranthus	28	Balance within yourself.
Star of Bethlehem	29	Ability to act from inner joy.

The Anahata Chakra

Centaury	4	Service.
Chicory	8	Overcoming distance.
Heather	14	Unconditional love.
Holly	15	Free-flowing love energy.
Honeysuckle	16	Living in the here and now.
Red chestnut	25	The ability to express true love.
Rock rose	26	Overcoming ego limitations.

The Vishuddha Chakra

Agrimony	1	Fusing thinking and feeling.
Mustard	21	Trusting your self, even in difficult times.
Wild oat	36	Communicating from your deepest soul.
Willow	38	Making space for creativity.

The Ajna Chakra

Beech	3	Tolerance.
Cerato	5	Following your inner guide.
Chestnut bud	7	Being open to learning from life.
Gentian	12	Acceptance.
Olive	23	Trusting cosmic harmony.
Vine	32	Accepting authority.
Walnut	33	Being able to listen to your inner voice.
White chestnut	35	An aid to meditation.

It is only sensible to use the Bach Flower Remedies in conjunction with the chakra work when you are concentrating for as much as two weeks on one chakra, though this does not mean that you have to work on that chakra every single day.

I usually combine two remedies for one chakra. I stop taking the remedy after two weeks or so, because by then the situation has usually changed anyway. I tend to think that if you use a particular remedy for more than two weeks in conjunction with the chakra work it starts to lose its power.[1]

There are many possibilities with these remedies, but you should use them quite sparingly. Like all remedies, they are only crutches, and it is surely more important to learn to grow without any crutches, finding the energy for the chakra work within ourselves rather than

relying on an external means of support. There are many
ways of asking your soul the right questions, but
unfortunately we are all sometimes so blocked, so blind
to what is really going on, that Bach Flowers or
homoeopathy can save hours of frustration. But is it
really helpful to cut corners? Is there such a thing as a
real short cut?

While I was at Findhorn I was part of a group which
worked with the Bach Flower Remedies — sometimes
we called them 'spiritual opium'!

Finally, some personal thoughts about the chakras.

I am always interested to hear of other people's
experience with chakra work, so please write to me if
you would like to tell me what it means for you. I have
now been working therapeutically with the chakras for
six years or so, and everything I can learn from others
helps me to heal the people I work with.

I have not written about the use of the pendulum in
relation to chakra work, mostly because I have never
been able to systematise my experiences with it. I have
come up with quite contradictory results whenever I
have tried to ascertain energy flow using a pendulum.
Sometimes it has moved in exactly the same way over a
closed chakra as over an open one. I think that this
maybe has something to do with the energy pattern
in my own chakras, but I have never been able to find
any systematic connection so far — maybe I am just
blind!

Another subject I have not touched on is the used of
glass pyramids and orgone accumulators, so beloved of
Wilhelm Reich. I have to admit to being rather sceptical
about their use in chakra work, and wary of the way
they work with a person's energy. It is difficult to
ascertain the appropriate amount of energy that a
person needs, and I suspect that the use of an energy

accumulator can easily lead to uncontrolled over-energising. On the other hand I see this technique as too passive. But I would like to know more about it, and maybe one day I shall change my mind.

I have similar reservations about working with pyramid power in chakra work, though I think the problem of controlling amounts of energy is easier. My experience is that pyramids exert a very subtle influence, and if you use them cautiously they can have a harmonising effect. Of all the experiments I have done with pyramids, the one which seemed to be the most harmonising was when I put tiny pyramids on all my chakras for a while, rather than working only on one.

Some years ago I lived for several weeks in Greece in a huge wooden pyramid, and when I did my chakra exercises there I was able to feel the energy flows in my body much more strongly. On the other hand, I was never able to sleep in the middle of the pyramid.

I have also worked with tuning forks. A truly amazing effect can be achieved if you set a tuning fork vibrating, then place it on your Sahasrara Chakra. Your whole skull seems to be filled with the sound, which appears to vibrate from inside your head. There is little effect with the same technique used at the other chakras.

If you work with tuning forks, the pitch of the note seems to matter. I experienced the best effects with the pitch of C sharp (which corresponds with the 'sa' pitch of the sitar[2], but you can also get a good effect using concert pitch A, which you can buy in any music shop.

I have written a lot in this book about harmony, and how with regular chakra work both our inner and outer harmony improve. At the beginning, however, it does not necessarily mean that we are aware of this growing harmony. When I started doing chakra work I was

quite puzzled when my dark side started coming up, and
I was using a great deal of energy to deal with it. Now I can
see that that tension is a very creative one. It is
this tension between wanting to be good and feeling
the evil inside me that still takes me deep into meditation. In the inner silence I fight to clear a space for
the good to fill.

With chakra work we are always fighting for paradise
— inner as well as outer — and we often overlook the
fact that we are actually destroying the paradise with
our powers of thought and reflection. Yet the effort
involved in working towards this paradise helps to
purify our mind like an alchemical transformation,
helping us to become more compassionate. Maybe this
is the highest aim of chakra work — to identify with
Avalokitesvara, the Buddha of compassion and mercy.

Chakra work is a path of self-understanding which
can affect the disciple quite profoundly. It has this in
common with any serious therapeutic path, and that
path is not without its sorrows. Working towards
harmony always leads through suffering and the pain of
paradise lost. It forces us to make difficult decisions,
yet it is precisely these decisions which lead to
profound change. As we grow we can see ourselves from
a greater height; see our energies as part of a greater
whole. This is precisely what is meant by that aspect of
the Sahasrara Chakra which enables us to see ourselves
from outside and above. This tension between reality
and ideal is exactly what produces the necessary
movement. The fixed condition of paradise allow little
movement.

I have come to understand this only after years of
working with the chakras. Maybe it isn't much to have
learned, but it has changed me profoundly. Sometimes I
am frightened of going further, but there is always only
the one real choice. To go on.

Gate, Gate, Paragate
Parasamgate
Bhodi svaha

Go, go, go beyond
Go beyond that beyond
All praise to the initiator

I hope that with this book I have given you some stimulation and useful information for setting out on the chakra work. I wish you joy with your work, for if there were no joy in it nobody would do it for long, and you need joy alongside your patience and determination!

"In your body is the mountain of Meru,
Surrounded by the seven continents.
There are streams, too,
Lakes, mountains, plains,
And the gods of the various regions.
There are prophets there,
Monks, and places of pilgrimage,
And above the ruling gods
There are stars, planets,
And the sun together with the moon;
And there are also the two cosmic powers,
The one that destroys and the one that creates;
And all the elements: ether,
Air and fire, water and earth.
Yes, all these things are within your body:
They exist in three worlds,
And all fulfil their ordered tasks
Around the mountain of Meru.
Only the one who knows this
Can become a true yogi"[3]

1. Chancellor, P.M. *Handbook of the Bach Flower Remedies* Daniel, 1985.

2. This is the sound of the annual vibration of the Earth in the 32nd octave, though for technical reasons we work one octave higher, with a tuning fork of 272.2Hz. This corresponds to the 'royal cubit', the measure used by the architects of the pyramids.

3. Siva Samhita 2, 1-5, translated by Varenne, Jean *Yoga and the Hindu Tradition* University of Chicago, 1977.

Glossary

AFFIRMATION
A positive statement which produces the power to turn what is spoken into reality.

AJNA
The Third Eye; the sixth chakra.

ANAHATA
The heart chakra; the fourth and central chakra.

ARDHA-MATSENDRAASANA
The twist: a classical yoga exercise.

ARKANA
An idea from the tarot (Cabala): the name of the 21 trumps of tarot.

ASANA
A body exercise in yoga; a yoga position.

ASSIMILATION
The biological concept of an organism's adaptation to its surroundings.

AVALOKITESVARA
The Buddha of mercy.

BHARATI-STHANA
'The dwelling place of the language of the gods': a name for the liberated throat chakra.

BHASTRA
A breathing technique (also used in rebirthing) where no pause is left between in-breath and outbreath, or between outbreath and inbreath.

BIJA
A female form of energy. Based on the Hindu Shakti (or form-giving) principle.

BINDU
A male form of energy. Based on the Hindu Shiva (or formless) principle.

BIOENERGETICS
A method of bodywork based theoretically on the work of Wilhelm Reich; practically on the work of Alexander Lowen. Bioenergetics works with ideas about energy similar to the concept of prana energy.

BUDDHA AMITHABA
The principle of the formless beginning, which says that enlightenment is impossible until all sensitive beings are enlightened. The Buddha of mercy brings the last sensitive being to enlightenment.

CHAKRAS
Energy centres in the body: there are seven main and innumerable minor chakras.

CHOD
A Tibetan text (from Hatha Yoga) about the chakra work.

DINERGY
The power that produces growth, based on the integration of opposites.

GESTALT THERAPY
A technique of humanistic psychology based on field theory, in which the here-and-now is vitally important, as is clear expression of feelings.

HALASANA
The plough; a classical yoga exercise.

HARA
A concept from Japanese Buddhism: the middle of your body around your navel.

HATHA YOGA
Literally 'sun and moon yoga'. A basic system of yoga that combines body, breathing and meditation exercises.

HOLOGRAM
A laser-produced picture in which any randomly chosen part contains the whole picture.

IDA
The female or yin aspect of the life force; one of the three channels up which the kundalini rises.

IYENGAR
Yoga following the contemporary Indian master Iyengar, who wrote classic works about bodywork and breathing.

JIN SHIN JYUTZU
A therapeutic technique in which the hands are used to connect parts of the body; body energies can thus be harmonised, leading to physiological and psychological healing.

KUNDALINI
The vital life force, symbolised by a snake; serpent power.

LAYA YOGA
A yoga system with the stress on chakra work.

LOTUS BLOSSOMS
A poetic and symbolic name for the seven main chakras as energy centres in the body.

MAITHUNA
In Tantra, the path of the fusion of male and female energies; corresponds with the Mysterium Conjuctionis of the alchemists.

MANIPURA
The navel or solar plexus chakra. The third chakra and centre of gravity of the body. Corresponds with the Japanese hara.

MANTRA
Holy or magical syllables, words or sentences, usually in Sanskrit or Tibetan. What they mean is of less importance than how they sound.

MATSYASANA
The fish: a classical yoga exercise.

MEDITATION
Different forms of centering and focusing your mind. The aim of every meditation is oneness.

MUDRA
Particular positions of the fingers which help centering and concentration during meditation.

MULADHARA
The base chakra; the lowest of the chakras.

NADA
Energy set free by the fusion of Shiva and Shakti; the place where duality is replaced by real understanding.

NADIS
'Yoga nerves' which channel energy through the body; some scientists see them as the meridians of acupuncture

PASCHIMOTTANASANA
The pliers; a classical yoga exercise.

PINGALA
The male or yang aspect of life energy; one of the three channels up which the kundalini rises.

PRANA
The basic energy that binds the psyche to the body.

PRANAYAMA
Breathing exercises in yoga.

PRATI PRASSAV
'In the service of progress'; meditation on your life story helping you to overcome resistance.

RAJAS
A concept from Indian philosophy which corresponds with the cardinal quality of astrology.

RAJA YOGA
A highly developed form of yoga based on long study of Hatha Yoga, the aim being to allow the kundalini to rise.

REBIRTHING
A method of bodywork which stresses breathing (see BHASTRA) together with affirmations.

RED TANTRA
In Red Tantra, sexuality is seen as a form of development and a manifestation of divine energy. During the ritual of sexual ecstasy, every limitation and illusion can be dissolved using Red Tantra concepts. In Red Tantra, woman and man meet as an embodiment of Shiva and Shakti, as goddess and god.

REFLEXOLOGY
The massage of certain points and areas of the soles of the feet, and sometimes also the area around the ankles. This regulates the functions of your vital organs.

SAHASRARA
The crown chakra or thousandfold lotus; the highest chakra.

SARVANGASANA
The shoulder stand; a classical yoga exercise.

SATTVA
A concept from Indian philosophy which corresponds with the mutable quality in astrology.

SKULD
The Third Norn in Germanic mythology.

SUKHAPADMA ASANA
An exercise from Red Tantra in which the woman and man touch each other's lower six chakras.

SUSHUMNA
The central aspect of life energy, connected with understanding and meditation; one of the three channels up which the kundalini rises.

SVADISTHANA
The sacral or sexual chakra; the second chakra.

SYNERGY
The working together of all
individual energies as a
whole (an equivalent of
'interference' in science),
forming a new quality of
energy in which the quality
transcends the sum of the
individual energies.

TAMAS
A concept from Hindu
philosophy, corresponding
with the fixed quality in
astrology.

VISHUDDHA
The throat chakra; the fifth
chakra.

YAMANTAKA
The Tibetan personification
of the one who overcomes
death.

YANG
The light or male archetype.

YIN
The dark or female arche-
type.

YONI ASANA
An exercise from Red
Tantra which uses sexuality
as a means of development.

About the Author

Klausbernd Vollmar was born on November 22nd, 1946, at Remscheid in West Germany. He studied German literature, linguistics and philosophy at Bochum University; was a Lecturer at the Goethe Institute in Finland; and won a scholarship from the Canada Council, lecturing at McGill University, Montreal. He had his own healing practice and advice centre in Solingen for a while, and has travelled widely in Asia and Africa. He now lives in Norfolk, where he gives individual advice and group workshops in chakra work.